THE CRYSTAL REIKI WORKBOOK

By Charles Lightwalker

and

Lyncara Aria Stewart

Revised in UK 2024

Email: charleslightwalker@yahoo.com

The Crystal Reiki Workbook

Author: Charles Lightwalker and Lyncara Aria Stewart

Copyright © 2024 Charles Lightwalker and Lyncara Aria Stewart

The right of Charles Lightwalker and Lyncara Aria Stewart to be identified as author of this work has been asserted by the author in accordance with section 77 and 78 of the Copyright, Designs and Patents Act 1988.

First Published in 2024

ISBN 978-1-83538-395-7 (Paperback)

Published by:
    Maple Publishers
    Fairbourne Drive, Atterbury,
    Milton Keynes,
    MK10 9RG, UK
    www.maplepublishers.com

A CIP catalogue record for this title is available from the British Library.

All rights reserved. No part of this book may be reproduced or translated in any form or by any means, electronic or mechanical, including photocopying, recording or by any information storage and retrieval system without written permission from the author.

This book is a memoir. It reflects the author's recollections of experiences over time. Some names and characteristics have been changed, some events have been compressed, and some dialogues have been recreated, and the Publisher hereby disclaims any responsibility for them.

Other Books written by Charles Lightwalker

Quantum Healing: The Synergy of Chiropractic and Reiki (co-authored with Pat Doughtery)

Crystal Reiki Workbook, co-authored with Lyncara Aria Stewart

Crystalline Reiki

Sound Healing with Tuning Forks

Advanced Sound Healing with Tuning Forks

Crystal and Gemstone Healing

Medical Intuition Handbook

Vibrational Yoga: Sonic Mysticism and Movement

Musings: Poetry, Philosophy and More

Bits N Pieces: Poetry & Ramblings

Animal Medical Intuition, co-authored with Lyncara Aria Stewart

Operating a Holistic Enterprise: Tips of the Trade

Books written by Lyncara Aria Stewart

Crystals for dreaming and their effects on the subconscious

Visions from the Crystal Skulls

Transmissions from the Crystal Skulls Oracle deck

Animal Medical Intuition, co-authored with Charles Lightwalker

Crystal Reiki Workbook, co-authored with Charles Lightwalker

All Rights Reserved

No part of this book may be reproduced in any form or by any means, without permission in writing from the authors.

Photography by Lyncara Stewart for Mintaka Mermaid media and cover picture copyright of Mintaka Mermaid.

DISCLAIMER

This information describes complementary health techniques that may help to facilitate the healing of one's physical, emotional, mental, and spiritual bodies. It is not to be used in place of medical care.

We do not diagnose or treat medical or psychological conditions or diseases nor do we encourage people to diagnose or treat medical conditions. As always, seek the care and advice of a professional health practitioner or veterinary surgeon.

The information provided in this manual is for educational purposes only.

All hands on healing with or without crystals and / or taken from this book is solely the responsibility of the persons involved and participants willing.

The authors cannot be held responsible for any illness, misunderstanding, loss, or misuse of the crystals and techniques in this book, used on oneself, others or animals.

CONTENTS

Other Titles by the Authors

Copyright and Disclaimer

Table of Contents

Introduction

A Brief History of Reiki

Chapter 1 Choosing Crystals

Chapter 2 Cleansing Crystals

Chapter 3 Programming Your Crystals

    Meditation

    Meditation Practices

    Healing

    Absent or Distance Healing

    Manifesting

Chapter 4 The Healing Properties of Gemstones

    Index of Gemstones

Chapter 5 Crystal Reiki Reflexology

Chapter 6 Crystal Reiki Massage

    Ketseuki Kokan Ho - Kekko Massage

    Byosen Scanning

Chapter 7 Star of David Crystal Reiki Configuration

Chapter 8 Four Directions Crystal Reiki Layout

Chapter 9 Crystal Reiki Relationship Configuration

Chapter 10 Twelve Quartz Crystal Reiki Configuration

Chapter 11 Crystal Reiki Grid Configuration

Chapter 12 Animals and Crystal Reiki

Afterthoughts and Closing Statements by the Authors

Reiki Lineage

Reiki Resources

Crystal Healing Accreditations

Reiki Resources

About the Author Charles Lightwalker

About the Co Author Lyncara Aria Stewart

Reiki Glossary of Terms

Final Afterthoughts

Closing Statement.

Introduction

In this Crystal Reiki Manual, we do not intend to say much about the Reiki symbols or the methods you learned in your weekend courses leading to your Reiki Master attunement. For the purposes of this manual, we will assume that you are already familiar with how to conduct a Reiki treatment.

We will assume that you may not know a great deal about crystal healing, so the first few chapters of this book will describe how to choose, cleanse and program your crystals.

It is very important for you to know and understand that quartz crystals will amplify all other healing energies. Thus, in addition to amplifying your inherent reiki energies, crystals will also amplify the energies of all other therapies including aromatherapy, massage, shiatsu, sound therapy, colour therapy, yoga etc. etc.

In this Crystal Reiki Workbook, we are going to share some very powerful ways of using crystals to amplify your reiki energies to the greater benefit of all your patients and clients.

It became apparent to us over the course of writing this book, that it was taking on a life of its own, and we found ourselves inspired to expand the contents of this book beyond mere Crystal Reiki into various realms of metaphysics and holism, the awareness of which will enhance your practice, and prepare you for the mysteries that are sure to make their appearances in the world and in your practices.

Describing the infinite with mere words is always difficult—there may be times when reading this material, that you may find it useful to take a break, and close your eyes to absorb the powerful and profound vibrational energies being presented.

We are always very happy to hear from you if you need any further information. Our crystal door is always open for you.

You can always send an email to: charleslightwalker@yahoo.com or mintakamermaid@gmail.com for Lyncara.

The Reiki Healing Precepts

Just for today I release all anger. Today feel no anger.

Just for today I release all worry. Have no worries.

I show gratitude for all my many blessings. Feel gratitude.

I earn my living with integrity. Show diligence in your undertaking.

I honour every living thing. Treat others with kindness.

A Brief History of Reiki

The history of Reiki is thought to go back many centuries back to the lost civilization of Atlantis. Some believe that Reiki was used during Atlantean times as a healing method using life force energy. And that this method was rediscovered by Dr. Mikao Usui at the end of the nineteenth century.

Dr. Usui had a spiritual experience, while suffering from Cholera, and it inspired him to study the ancient teachings handed down by his ancestors, and after many years of study Usui discovered references to an ancient form of healing , continued research revealed symbols and methods on how to practise the art of hands on healing using life force energy. After several years of practising this method, Usui felt he needed a deeper, more spiritual understanding into how to create a healing system that utilises chi energy.

Dr. Usui decided to go to the holy mountain Kurama, he left the monastery he was living in and walked to the top of the mountain, sat down and meditated for 21 days. On the 21st day, Usui was hit with a bright light on his forehead. The bright light knocked him unconscious and while in this unconscious and altered state of awareness, he had a vision of sacred symbols and hand positions that were to be used in the healing process. After regaining consciousness, Usui , started back down the mountain to share his insights, and returned to the monastery. On his way down he stumbled and injured his foot, bleeding and in pain, he instantly placed his hands on his foot, the pain and bleeding immediately stopped. A short distance further he stopped at a village to eat some food. The young woman who served him his food was in pain and her face was swollen from a toothache, Usui asked if he could place his hands on her face, she agreed, and within a moment her pain vanished and her swelling disappeared. Upon his arrival back at the sanctuary, he found the Abbott in bed suffering, in pain with arthritis. So once again he placed his hands on the Abbott, and was able to alleviate the pain and suffering. He knew this was a sign.

Usui saw this as a gift from God, and that he was now guided to be a healer. The Abbott suggested that Usui go to the slums of Kyoto to heal the beggars of their affiliations. It was during this time, Usui realised that one must not only heal the body, but must also heal the mind and spirit of the person and create a healthy and balanced life. A complete Healing. Upon further meditations and visions, Usui formed the five principles of Reiki with a focus on gratitude, a focus on work and balance.

The remainder of Usui's life was spent healing, teaching and expanding the Usui Shiki Royoho method of healing. Dr. Usui had nineteen students he had trained to the Master level, and upon his death, Dr. Chujiro Hayashi was chosen as the Grandmaster.

Dr, Hayashi was responsible for training another sixteen Reiki Masters,and created a set formula for the attunement process. Dr Hayashi, was also a qualified physician and retired Marine commander, he wrote extensively on the Reiki healing system, until he left his body in 1940, after a ceremony to release his spirit from his body. But before he left his body he gathered all his students, and named Madam Hawajo Takata as his successor. Madame Takata, was the first woman ever attuned as a Reiki Master (1938) Madame Takata, went on to train twenty-two Reiki Masters before her death in 1980. At the time of her death, two Grandmasters were installed to carry on the work, one was Phyllis Lei Furumoto, her Granddaughter, and the other was Dr. Barbara Weber. They worked together for about a year and then each one went separate ways and created separate organisations.

Chapter 1: Choosing Your Crystals

All crystals and gemstones vibrate on their own individual frequency. In that respect they are similar to human beings; we also vibrate on a particular unique frequency.

We have all had the experience of meeting a perfect stranger and either liking that person immediately or feeling an inexplicable antipathy towards them.

To fall in romantic love is a beautiful and wonderful experience - the coming together of two minds, two spirits and two physical bodies, both vibrating on the same beautiful, loving frequency!

The way we choose crystals and gemstones is similar to the way we choose our friends and lovers. It is essential that the crystals and gemstones we choose and use should 'vibrate' on a frequency as near as possible to our own. As you develop and become more aware of your Crystal Reiki energies, you will intuitively find it easy to know which crystals you should use in your therapeutic work.

The techniques for choosing crystals and gemstones vary from person to person but they all normally include the following:

1) Close your eyes and quietly meditate for a few moments. Then open your eyes and pick up the first crystal or gemstone to which your eye becomes naturally drawn.

2) Run your hand (either your left or right hand depending upon which you prefer to use) over all the crystals and gemstones available for selection. You will soon discover that one crystal or gemstone will 'stick' to your hand as if it is 'tacky' or surrounded with glue. This is your crystal or gemstone; the one which you need to use.

You may feel the crystal emitting a vibration or a sensation in your hand, or even 'showing' you a colour, image or giving you a certain 'sense' or feeling. These are strong connections to crystals and a good indicator of co-creating for powerful crystal energy!

(Lyncara) - *I advise any person who feels such a strong effect or download from a crystal to apply time to work with it and not shy away from the energy and effects given from the crystal. Powerful healing and energy work can be gained from such instances and connection to the crystal.*

3) Intuitively you will 'know' which stone is 'right' for you! You may feel as if it is jumping up and down shouting, "Me! Me! Me! Choose Me!" Or you might sense, or even 'see', a strong crystalline white light radiating from the crystal and attracting you like a magnet.

4) Should you happen to be a competent dowser, you may be able to select the most appropriate crystal or gemstone by using your own preferred dowsing technique.

Sometimes it feels as if your stones are actually choosing you.

(Charles) *This has often happened to me. All my most powerful and energised quartz crystals have arrived on my doorstep (so to speak) for a particular purpose and have a special reason for wanting me to work with them. Normally they have been either absolutely free or have cost me very little money.*

Should you wish to choose a Quartz crystal or a gemstone for one of your friends who, perhaps, lives some distance away, follow exactly the same principles as if you were choosing a personal crystal or gemstone for yourself but on this occasion visualise, as strongly as possible, an image of your friend in your mind's eye.

With a little practice you will soon discover that it is easy to select just the right Quartz crystal or gemstone for any of your friends who are unable to choose their stones in person for themselves. Always go by your first impressions, and your first intuitive instinct. Too much thought and hesitation will only lead to you becoming confused and uncertain!

(Lyncara) I have watched many people choose and become connected to crystals over the years. They can spend many minutes or even hours browsing and hesitating over a crystal, especially if they have no knowledge or experience working with crystals. It is almost certain that a person will settle for the first or initial crystal they picked up or found themselves drawn to! I believe that on a subconscious level, the connection of the crystal deva to us and its workings on our energy field is intrinsically linked. Irrespective of the crystal's material and compounds, it will naturally take on a personal healing facilitation on some level.

If you are torn between two crystals or remain uncertain, close your eyes, pick up one or both crystals at a time and quietly sit until you 'feel' the crystal that has the strongest effect on you. This can come in the form of vibration, tingling, evoking feelings and emotions, images and colours or words coming to you. Sometimes taking away the visual concept and allowing other senses to take over can be a great way of choosing the right crystal and expanding on your connection to crystalline energies. Some crystals can have a powerful effect.

(Lyncara) I have a Quartz Crystal Skull that came to me somewhat unexpectedly. Upon my first meditation with it, it kept showing me a high mountain scape with many snowy peaks and projecting words to me in a different language. I had no idea what it was saying and at first I thought it was trying to give me a name. Upon further research it quickly became apparent that the skull had given me a complete poem, in language I had never heard or seen before! As it turns out, it was made from Himalayan Quartz and it had in fact downloaded to me, a Tibetan prayer! (I talk more about this experience, prayer and workings with this skull and other skulls in my book, 'Visions from the Crystal Skulls')

Although more and more retail outlets are now selling crystals and gemstones there are still many towns and cities throughout the world where it is difficult, if not impossible, to purchase crystals and gemstones in person.

For many people, the only real opportunity they have to select a crystal or gemstone personally is to attend one of the regular workshops and seminars conducted by holistic healers such as ourselves. At every workshop and seminar there are always a large selection of crystals, gemstones, and books available for purchase.

In cases where people simply cannot find crystals or attend a crystal healing seminar, it is still possible to help them find good stones. What we do in this case is match the vibration of a crystal to the vibration of their or a piece of their correspondence—even an email. From all the feedback we receive it would certainly appear that this method works well in most instances.

As you develop your Crystal Reiki healing energies, you will soon find that you will easily be able to help your long-distance clients in much the same way!

Chapter 2 : Cleansing Crystals

Having chosen your crystal or gemstone (by whichever method you may have used) it is now very important that you cleanse it.

Quartz crystals and gemstones often attract all kinds of vibrations, negative as well as positive. The stones are always open to receiving impressions from everyone and everything around them!

The crystal or gemstone you have just selected may well have travelled many thousands of miles before coming to you, and it may well have acquired some negative energies and vibrations in its long and arduous journey to find you!

Therefore, before starting to use your crystal or gemstone for any healing purpose it is important that you first remove all of these unwanted negative 'vibrations' and disharmonious energies before you commence to use your stone for healing purposes.

You must do everything you can to ensure that only the most pure and natural remain within your stone.

The cleansing method you use is always a matter of personal choice, and is usually dependent upon the crystal structure and composition, but we have found the following methods to be very successful:

1) Hold your crystal or gemstone in either your left or right hand (according to personal preference) and say these words: "I will and command that this crystal or gemstone be self-cleansing." As you repeat these words quietly or aloud, you can also accompany them with visualising a cleansing, radiant white light surrounding and penetrating through the crystal and removing and dissolving any unwanted energy, leaving only the natural and pure energies in the crystal.

2) Water is a wonderful universal cleanser. Hold your crystal or gemstone under cold flowing water from a stream, river, waterfall, leave in rainfall or hold under the tap (cold water only. Never use hot water!) and, again, visualise all the negative energies and 'vibrations' being washed away and leaving behind only the pure and natural energies behind.

When drying your crystal and gemstone after cleansing in water never attempt to dry them using a towel or cloth. Always allow your crystals and gemstones to dry naturally - preferably from the rays of the sun if suitable! If you have a crystal that is prone to fading in sunlight, find a place out of direct sunlight to allow them to air dry in a breeze or as naturally as possible in the warmth of your own home.

For the crystals that may not be suitable for sunlight all the time, you can leave them to dry naturally under moonlight instead.

The sun, of course, is always a very powerful energizer and should be used whenever possible. Certain crystals energetically thrive in a little sunlight and some crystals are prone to becoming brittle and fading. If you do wish to use solar energy for crystals, please use discretion on the material of the crystal and the time for which you leave the crystals in the sun. Crystals can become very hot in the sunlight after a short period of time and you want the crystal to remain in good condition for longevity. Remember crystals are unearthed from the ground and so do not need a long time in the sun and elements to cleanse and charge.

3) Immerse your crystal or gemstone of suitable composition in salt water. You can use the ocean if it is preferable and dry as indicated above. However, it is recommended that you do not leave salt on the crystal and leave it in sunlight. You would be better rinsing the crystal with fresh water afterward and especially if choosing the sunlight method.

4) Bury your crystals and gemstones under the earth in your garden. Our planet Earth consists of at least one third quartz and the very strong and powerful magnetic energy field in the actual earth will 'cleanse' your crystals and gemstones of all their negativity very effectively.

N.B. If you own a dog, be very careful! Dogs find it great fun to dig up crystals.

5) Place your crystal or gemstone on a large Quartz crystal cluster or Selenite slab for a few hours. The very strong crystalline energies present within the cluster will soon neutralise any negative energy that may be in your crystals and gemstones. Selenite has a more gentle energy but quickly returns crystals to a balanced and cleansed condition.

Even though Quartz, Selenite and Garnet are considered self cleansing, it is still wise if using plates or larger clusters to attend to them by smudging with Palo Santo, Sage, Copal or another form of cleansing you see to be appropriate.

6) Frequency can be used to move energy from the crystal. You can use a Singing bowl or tuning fork to do this. The fork or bowls frequency cleanses, energises and realigns the crystal's optimal vibration. This method can also emit the frequencies of the crystal outward if used in sound baths, so it would be important to use this method twice or cleanse the crystal beforehand if using on others. There is a specific Crystal Tuning Fork, emitting at 4096 Hz used for activating and cleansing which is to be toned and moved around the crystal or toned and the stem gently placed on the crystal for a few seconds.

IMPORTANT: Please note the need for suitable cleansing and charging methods for the crystal material in question and take into regard its formations and finishes. Listed below are factors to take into consideration.

Before your choice of cleansing and care needed for the crystal. The material differences that factor into this are:

<u>Raw and polished form</u> - Raw and polished form can affect the way you cleanse a crystal, a crystal you would not submerge in water usually in its natural or raw form can sometimes be used in this method if tumbled or polished.

<u>Crystals that are water and salt soluble</u> - Are the crystals likely to dissolve or erode if exposed to water or this method is used over time? Some popular crystals that are water soluble are: Celestite, Selenite, Fluorite, Turquoise, Lapis Lazuli, Lepidolite, Hematite, Apophyllite, Apatite.

<u>Crystals that fade in sunlight</u> - Is the crystal likely to fade or get brittle in sunlight if this method is used over time? Popular crystals that fade in prolonged sun exposure are Amethyst, Citrine, Rose quartz, Labradorite, Apatite, Beryls, Opals.

<u>Toxic mineral compositions and inclusions</u> - Some crystals contain toxic elements that we become exposed to through handling (usually in raw form) or when they are exposed to water, broken or crushed.

Popular crystals and minerals of toxicity are: Malachite, Azurite, Chrysocolla, Pyrite, Iolite, Bumblebee Jasper - whilst the stones listed are safe to wear and hold in fully polished form, anything with high copper content should not be used direct in elixirs and essences and used with indirect method only. (Always wash your hands after handling toxic minerals or crystals).

<u>Delicate and Fragile crystals</u> - Celestite, Kyanite, Desert Rose Selenite, Halite (All water soluble).

If you are unsure then a method such as visualisation, reiki, smudging and vibration may be best.

As a rule, anything less than 6 on the Moh hardness scale must be judged according to material compounds. The Mohs hardness scale is a measure of resistance, scratching and abrasion. The hardness of a mineral is determined by observing whether its surface is scratched by a substance of known or defined hardness.

This list is in no way extensive and it would be wise to learn and acquire new knowledge about any crystals you may choose to work with so you can care for them accordingly.

It is also recommended that you do not submerge your crystals in water for long periods of time. If needed for elixir's or essences the indirect method can be used.

Elixir's indirect method is having two bowls or containers, the inner bowl or container would hold your water and the outer would be used for placing Crystals so they do not come into contact with the water but the energies can transfer to the water. Alternatively a crystal can simply be left next to a glass of water or the container holding the elixir water.

The science of making a crystal elixir or essence with this method is that water is a conductor and a water cell can be programmed just like a crystal. It will retain the information or energy exposed to it and amplify it.

Elixirs are great to drink and essences can be used to spray in rooms, auric fields and over yourself and the client before, during and after a healing session.

Chapter 3: Programming your Crystals

All Quartz crystals and gemstones will respond to the 'intent' of your own personal will, whether in word, in thought, in mantra or in practice.

Now you have made an initial connection to your crystal by being drawn to it, ask some simple questions. How does it make you feel? What was apparent to you in your life when the crystal made its appearance? Perhaps it already has a meaning or dedication towards its intended use or is designed to work for you on or in a specific manner. Use this information in your connection with the crystal to help you decide what to infuse with the programming.

Sometimes it is beneficial to see the crystal as a being and let it show you its effects, as this can give subconscious information to us. Let the crystal breathe and allow it to first be multifaceted and multi functional. Then we can confirm its use and programme as necessary. The crystal shares energy itself, therefore, after cleansing, if you do not feel the need to programme a particular crystal, then it isn't necessary at that time. Practise awareness with crystals, they are vibrationary tools, akin to a living being. Programming does not alter or change the vibration of the crystal as such, but creates a bond for the set workings to be undertaken through the intent.

By simply wishing or visualising the crystalline energy to be used in a particular way, you will find that it happens! It really is that simple.

Quartz crystals are usually 'programmed' for the following purposes: Meditation, Healing, Distance Healing, and Manifesting. Let's look at each of these in turn.

Meditation

Throughout the world, every day of the week, every minute of every day, countless thousands of people are practising some form of meditation. Although each person finds solace and comfort meditating in their own particular way, we submit that by holding a Quartz crystal or an Amethyst in your hand while meditating, anybody will enhance and enrich the spiritual depths of their meditative experience.

A Quartz or Amethyst crystal will enable you to undertake a new and wondrous journey to the inner recesses of your soul. Unknown pathways, hitherto uncharted, will open up before you.

A new dimension of self-expression will rise to the surface and expand your inner consciousness and awareness.

The Amethyst, of course, is well known for being able to relieve mental and physical stress and tension. It is the stone emitting inner peace and tranquillity, the stone of sublime relaxation.

Every member of your meditation circle or group should have their very own piece of Quartz or Amethyst to hold throughout the meditation session.

With the passing of time, people meditating with a crystal will gradually become aware that their breathing has become deeper and more rhythmical, and may feel that they have entered a new world of inner peace and harmony.

All meditation rooms would greatly benefit from placing large Quartz crystals at all four corners of the room with their single-terminated points directed towards the centre of the room. These crystals should ideally be placed either on the floor or affixed to the corners of the ceiling.

Each of the four Quartz crystals in the meditation room should be 'programmed' to project gentle, loving, relaxing, and crystalline reiki energy towards all those present within the Meditation group. The Quartz crystals will then generate a field of positive crystalline reiki energy to surround everyone in the room.

Moreover, in addition to having every member of the meditation group hold their own individual amethyst or Quartz crystal, a large Amethyst or Quartz crystal cluster should also be placed in the middle of the group. This large cluster should then be 'programmed' to release beautiful cosmic crystalline reiki energies into every corner of the room.

It is very important that one member of the meditation group should be nominated to look after the group's Amethyst or Quartz crystal cluster - and to make certain that it is properly cleansed, dedicated and programmed.

If you hold your crystal or Amethyst when meditating with music, you will often experience some amazing effects being produced. On some occasions you might even be able to see the music in terms of its colour and shape.

Even just listening to a piece of music while holding a Quartz crystal or Amethyst—and not necessarily trying to meditate consciously—you will find the depth of the listening experience greatly enriched by the crystal's presence.

Whenever harmonious music is being played in the presence of your crystal or amethyst, the mood and thoughts of the composer become deeply embedded within the very heart of the crystal and if you 'listen' to the crystal afterwards, with your inner ear, you will often be able to pick up the esoteric resonance and meaning of the music itself.

You may use your crystal or Amethyst in many ways when meditating. Do not be afraid to experiment and try new methods. Listen to what your crystal is saying and try to respond accordingly. You will find the results truly amazing and very worthwhile.

Some recommended Crystal Meditation Practices

Now you are ready to try your own Crystal Reiki meditation. I would suggest that you hold either a piece of natural Quartz crystal—or a piece of Amethyst—in whichever hand feels best.

Now, lie or sit in a comfortable position. Close your eyes, relax and breathe slowly. Say a prayer of protection, perhaps the Great Invocation, or even your own impromptu prayer. Or, perhaps, draw some of the Reiki Symbols towards you, to envelop your physical body.

Hold your crystal between both your hands and locate the opening to the crystal. Do this by slowly and intuitively rubbing your thumbs and fingers across the faces of the crystal, moving slowly from one face to the other.

The objective is to find a spot where your thumb or finger sticks like glue onto the crystal. This is your opening into the crystal and into the crystal energies.

Breathe slowly and deeply relax your mind and body. Relax all your muscles starting with your feet and gradually working your way up through the rest of your body till you arrive at your head.

First exhale and then inhale and exhale again, allowing yourself to relax and rid yourself of all internal stress within your body. Allow your body to sink deeper and deeper into the floor. Let go; hold nothing back. Allow your head, and now your neck, to relax, and continue letting go of all tension.

Relax your throat and then your shoulders, letting the burdens fall off them onto the floor. Let your arms and your fingers relax, feel the tension being released.

Now relax your chest, back, spine and abdomen; breathe slowly and deeply. Inhale, exhale, allow the tension to fall off your body and onto the floor.

You do not need this tension anymore! You have no further use for it. Now your waist, buttocks, pelvis, thighs, knees, calves, and feet; relax each of them in turn. Let all the tension go. Again, breathe slowly and deeply, inhaling, exhaling.

Now bring your awareness to the crystal between your hands. Turn your attention to the entry point into the crystal and merge with the crystal and with your breath. Together, exhale, inhale and focus on your entry point and then exhale again, merging and merging more fully into the crystal.

Release your expectations, your thoughts, and your personality, and surrender to your own inner being. Let all the inner tension slowly rise to the surface and let it all fall from your body to the floor.

Let us now fully merge with the crystal. Let us inhale, exhale, inhale, focusing on the entry point. Exhale. Feel the crystal energies engulfing you, enveloping you, surrounding you.

Allow your senses to become very acute: your sense of touch and taste, smell, hearing, and sight, as you begin touching the wall of the crystal.

Notice the temperature, taste the crystal energies, listening, listening for any sounds, voices, noises.

Expand your vision.

Look around to see what it feels like to be within a crystal, to be within these exquisite energies.

Allow yourself to breathe deeply, to relax, to heal. Become aware of your every breath and see how relaxed your whole body has now become. There is nothing to do; there is only to be and to feel these healing energies.

Breathe the love into you, take it in. Allow the healing to go deeper, and deeper within, into your core, the very essence of your being, your soul and your spark of divine life.

When you have received all the healing, and released all the tension from your physical and mental bodies; when you have received all the healing energy that you need, gently, slowly, feel your consciousness being pulled to the wall of the crystal.

You will recognize that you are very relaxed and stress-free, and that as you return to your every-day existence you will be a changed person because of this profound experience of deep love, this new understanding that is now yours, that has gone so deep within your soul and the very essence of your own divinity.

Notice how you are feeling and recognize that at any time you can return to the crystal energies. Now, however, it is time to release yourself from the crystal. Leave as you enter; exhale, inhale, focus on releasing from the crystal; exhale, letting go, relaxing, breathing evenly and less deeply.

Withdraw yourself from the crystal, slowly, once again inhaling deeply, and focus on receding further from the crystal. Exhale, withdrawing your energies, and then place your crystal by your side.

Say a prayer of thanks for all that you have received, and slowly begin drawing your arms over your head in a lazy stretch. Begin moving your fingers and toes. Now you are back in your own room.

There are many other forms of crystal reiki meditation that you might like to try.

For example, turn out all the lights in your meditation room and sit in a comfortable chair in front of a table with a lighted white candle on it.

Then, place a Quartz crystal upright in front of you with the lighted candle behind it. Make sure the crystal is at your eye-level. Look at the flame of the candle through your crystal and gradually become aware of your breathing. Breathe in, breathe out, breathe in, breathe out, slowly and steadily relaxing.

Continue to gaze into the flame, aware of your body, breathing slowly and rhythmically, becoming more and more relaxed.

If you find that random ideas and thoughts keep passing through your mind, allow them to come and go gently; let them be free to roam. Keep gazing into the flame and become still within yourself. Slow down your breathing and let your whole-body metabolism become calm and peaceful.

Try to do a crystal reiki meditation at least once per day for twenty minutes. You will soon find that your whole being becomes more calm, peaceful and relaxed!

Healing

Once you have chosen your Quartz crystal, and have cleansed and dedicated it, you are ready to begin using it for healing purposes.

It is very important to note, however, that for best results your Quartz crystal should only be used for either healing or meditation. Not for both!

The vibrations and energies used in healing and meditation are very different and to use the same Quartz crystal for both purposes could result in the dissipation of the crystal's unique energies.

We suggest using Quartz for healing and Amethyst for meditation. Even though both are primarily Quartz, Amethyst has Iron and other trace elements that when irradiated, give Amethyst its colour. The colour is associated with the third eye chakra and therefore more so used in meditative and perceptive uses.

In their passive state, quartz crystals are only 'tools'. By themselves they can only be described as passive; but when they become activated by the human mind, they can become extremely powerful indeed.

Each one of us, as members of the human species, possesses an inherent healing energy. In most people, of course, this healing ability lies totally dormant and inactive.

But when we possess the knowledge that enables us to channel our own healing energy and reiki energies, we can, with the help of our Quartz crystal friends, amplify this healing power. The resulting energy that we create in conjunction with that of our crystals may be used for many positive healing purposes.

Even if you should not wish to practise as a Crystal Reiki Therapist yourself there are still plenty of opportunities for you to use your quartz crystals together with your reiki healing energies to heal your family and friends.

If you do treat clients, the following guide-lines may prove helpful:

1) At the beginning of the healing session, you should hold your Quartz crystal in whichever hand feels right to you; and calmly attune yourself to the inner energies of your Quartz crystal. You will probably experience energies 'throbbing' within your hand.

2) Direct the single-terminated end of your healing quartz crystal towards your client and gently move the crystal around the perimeter of their whole body in a clockwise direction.

As you do this, at the same time visualise a blue-white crystalline light emanating from the apex of the client's body and flowing towards the client and surrounding them. Do this several times. This will help to strengthen the electro-magnetic field of energy around the physical body of the client.

3) Direct the single-terminated end of the Quartz crystal directed towards that part of the client's body which you believe or sense to be most in need of healing.

4) Visualise, as strongly as possible, a lovely blue-white light emanating from the apex of your crystal once again and direct this light, like a laser beam, to that part of the client's body where you feel that the healing is most needed. This lovely blue white becomes stronger and brighter as the energy between the crystal and your client slowly begins to intensify.

The crystal healing session itself may, in theory at any rate, last any length of time, but intuitively you will become aware of when the time is right to bring the session to an end.

5) To finish the crystal healing treatment session, you should visualise the blue-white light gently flowing back into your Quartz crystal. Once more you should direct and project the healing energies around the perimeter of your client's body in a clockwise direction. Then allow your client to relax for a few minutes.

Many clients regularly fall fast asleep so it is very important that you bring them back to the present in as relaxed a manner as possible.

Whenever practical it is best for your client not to have to drive a car for some time after the crystal healing session as the client often becomes so de-stressed that they may 'space out' that it can take considerable time for them to reorient themselves!

(Charles) *While I often do discuss a client's medical history with them before offering any form of treatment, from my own personal experience I have found that it is not always necessary to know, in advance, what is medically wrong with my client.*

My own personal belief is that all dis-ease occurs purely as a result of an imbalance of our normal bodily vibrations. Therefore, whatever health condition from which we may suffer, however serious or mild, whether it be cancer, multiple sclerosis, tumours or simply a dose of influenza or the common cold, the basic treatment remains much the same.

All that is really necessary is that the disharmonious or imbalanced vibrations be re-harmonized, reenergized and re-balanced.

This may, at first sight, appear to be an oversimplification but years of experience has shown me that all too often we can over-complicate our diagnoses.

The main difference between allopathic medicine and natural medicine is that allopathic medicine treats symptoms whilst natural medicine concentrates upon finding the root cause of the health problem.

Simply put, if we can discover the originating cause or imbalance of any health condition or dis-ease, we can, by using our Reiki Crystal Healing techniques, rebalance all the vibrations which are out of alignment. We can then effect a cure or, at the very least, a gradual improvement in the client's overall health!

(Lyncara) *In my experience with clients, it is not always enough to 'think the body well'. As much as the brain is a powerful tool, you can not lie to your body or the information that cells hold, you must influence them through physical and mental health. That is why it is functional to use Crystal Reiki techniques as a full body system for mind, body and energy, and for you and the client to connect these systems harmoniously and in equilibrium before internal and external, mind and body, inner and outer energies can fully stabilise, integrate and allow deep healing to occur.*

The body must 'feel' safe. In order for this, the nervous system must be regulated. This can take time for some clients as they are learning to reprogram the nervous system and trust themselves and their intuition again in the process. This process can help one in remaining consistent with their healing and energy systems going forward.

The body adapts to protect from chronic stress, when limited capacity and resources are available or given over a period of time, this can come in the form of mental and physical traumas and long term states of stress, deficiencies, chronic pain etc and therefore the body shows more symptoms as it tries to communicate its needs, after ignoring or being unaware of the body's needs for so long, it is important to revisit brain and body connection, rebuilding trust and intuition and physically bringing in more support for all the body systems. Designating time to be fully present with the ongoing process and sessions can help one in finding and keeping more in balance to support the body, mind and energetic systems.

Crystal Healing and Crystal Reiki can facilitate shifts in areas of the body and allow the client to connect to areas that require awareness or energy healing work to bring into balance throughout the body systems.

You may also, of course, use your Quartz crystal for self-healing purposes. All you have to do is to direct the single-terminated end of your crystal towards the appropriate part of your own body and, as you did before when treating your client, visualise a lovely blue-white light radiating from the apex of your crystal, like a laser beam, into your own body.

Crystal Healing is one of the most powerful and effective methods of re-balancing, re-energizing, and re-harmonizing every part of the physical and mental bodies of either yourself or of your client. Quartz is known as the master healer and is a very powerful and efficient crystal as a tool for healing.

Absent or Distant Healing

Quartz crystals are often used successfully in all forms of absent, or distant healing. Whether you are three miles, three hundred miles, three thousand miles, or thirteen thousand miles away from your client, Crystal Reiki healing can prove most effective.

For best results it is recommended that the quartz crystals you use for absent healing purposes are used solely for absent healing and for no other purpose.

It is only necessary to have the name of the person who wishes to receive absent healing. Absent Healing, using the unique power of Quartz crystals, can work solely on the name vibration alone.

All you have to do is visualise the crystalline energy pulsating within your absent healing Quartz crystal being projected towards your client, wherever he or she may live. Your Quartz crystal will do the rest!

If, however, you should have in your possession an actual photograph of your client, you can conduct your Crystal Reiki workings over the photograph or, if you have already met the person and therefore know what they look like, just hold your crystal in your hands and visualise, as strongly as possible, the crystalline energy surrounding the client.

In addition, it is very helpful after the absent healing session has been completed, to place your absent healing Quartz crystal on a photograph of your client; this assists the amplification of the crystalline energy which is being projected by the crystal towards your client.

You may find it useful to use a Master absent healing quartz crystal for all your absent healing treatments. If you are asked to do an absent healing, inscribe the client's name and relevant details in an absent healing book, and then place your Master absent healing Quartz crystal on top of this book with the program that every name entered in the book will receive healing from the crystalline energies, each according to his or her needs. It is useful to establish a set time, such as 10:00 pm every evening, for people to link up with your Master absent healing Quartz crystal.

Manifesting

(Charles) *Very simply, manifesting is a method of programming your Quartz crystal to help your subconscious mind bring into being something tangible in your life that you may need. Notice that I use the word need not want. There is a very big difference!*

Before you proceed with any form of manifesting it is extremely important that you examine your conscience and decide exactly what it is you wish to achieve. Decide, in as much precise detail as possible, whatever it is you need to acquire.

To avoid dissipating the crystalline energies, as already stated previously, it is most essential that you only use your chosen crystal for manifesting purposes only!

Let me repeat once again. Need, not want, should be your main criteria! For example, we might all say that we want to win the lottery jackpot of $10,000,000, but that is most definitely a want, not a need!

There was once a man who desperately desired a Cadillac. He could think of nothing else. So, he used his Quartz crystal to manifest one.

He visualised a Cadillac for days and days, until, at last, his dearest wish was granted. A Cadillac went out of control, skidded, and crashed through the window of the front room of his house!! This is a classic instance of not making it clear exactly what it was he wanted to manifest.

So be warned!

(Lyncara) Manifestation can work similar to intent, for change and betterment of self, habits, thought process, to make physical changes occur and forward movement and momentum. If we know better, we do better, physically and mentally.

The idea that what you see is seeking you, by resonance and matching frequency is partially true, frequency can and does attract the same to a certain degree but remember, you already emit a frequency on a base level, and it does not pre determine what you attract to you in manifesting. You cannot change this frequency as such but can learn to co-create with your mind, expanding this energy and into existence by engaging internally and externally with purpose, physical action, effort, consistency and taking action alongside the visualisation process of materialisation.

While manifestation embraces some proven concepts about self-efficacy, goal achievements and materialisations, it is important to clearly define what you need and the defining steps you may need to do to help aid your manifestation desires and achieve the goals and outcomes that you wish to see. Matching effort, input and output to succeed in physical and mental manifesting is key. (You would not want to be disappointed just visualising something that may indeed come through some mental manifestation but didn't fully transpire due to a bit of physical effort you also needed to input). Adding specific visualisation, imagining the idea of it already being so, along with the practical steps to get you closer to the end result is the magic recipe for trying to create success in manifesting. Being realistic, practical and taking small steps will aid you in your practice and manifestation journey until it becomes second nature!

By activating the heart space and remaining authentic to ourselves, we naturally raise our energy and expand our own frequency and by doing so we open up and bring to ourselves the illumination of our own inner awareness, hopes, dreams and desires to our highest self and potential.

Now, make yourself comfortable in an easy chair and let us begin to start manifesting your innermost needs.

First, hold your Quartz crystal in front of you, with both hands. Stare at it intently and visualise yourself entering into the crystal through a door cut into the crystal.

Once through this door you will find yourself in a long narrow hall. At the end of this hall is a green door inscribed with the words "MANIFESTING ROOM" written upon it.

Open the door of this Manifesting Room, step inside and look around. The walls are solid gold; the floor is green; the ceiling is studded with millions of precious gemstones, sparkling with all the colours of the rainbow. The room is filled with a warm, rich feeling of abundance.

Bring into your mind a complete and exact image of whatever it is you wish to manifest. Visualise as much detail as possible; concentrate as hard as you possibly can and imagine that you actually possess whatever it is you are manifesting. You are extremely happy and relaxed, secure in the knowledge that your need has been met.

Take your time; five, ten, or even fifteen minutes, it doesn't matter. Then, when you have finished, slowly walk back out of the Manifesting Room, closing the door firmly behind you.

Walk back along the hall and step outside of the crystal. Take a large deep breath, relax your body and when you feel comfortable, open your eyes.

Do your manifesting at least twice per day (morning and evening) until your need has been fulfilled.

Remaining consistent in thoughts and thought patterning, adapting to a more positive or abundance mindset may be beneficial for some. Perhaps daily activities and actions that draw you closer to your desired outcome would be a better course of action, be it remaining in a balanced headspace, or energy throughout the day, maintaining clarity of thought and actions, even searching and looking for opportunities or resonances that bring you closer to your desired result.

Sometimes manifestation isn't about big thoughts, or desires, it can be about maintaining a daily sense of self, mind or physical action. Manifestation can be about the very practical, simple things in our lives, it is all about how you show up for yourself everyday and how you want to create the happiest life you can for yourself.

We are not always in control of the things that happen to us and for us but we can take action and accountability on the things that we can control and learn to harmonise and balance ourselves and our life, daily and for the bigger picture.

Chapter 4: The Healing Properties of Gemstones

Although no guarantee of any radical or permanent cure can be made, there have been many occasions when the crystals and gemstones referred to in this book have helped considerably to bring about a positive improvement in many different diseases and health conditions.

The most effective way to use any crystal or gemstone for healing purposes is to wear it as close to the skin as possible.

Some women seem to 'hide' their gemstones within the deep inner recesses of their bras but most people prefer to wear their chosen gemstone around their neck on silver- or gold-plated chains.

In addition to the healing energies of the crystal or gemstone being able to penetrate the subtle body more easily, the crystal/gemstone pendant is a beautiful piece of jewellery, and is always aesthetically pleasing to the eye.

Remember - a stone of beauty is a joy forever!

Crystals and gemstones may, if so desired, be held in your hand whilst you are watching Television during the evening, or whilst you are reading a favourite book or magazine.

You may also place your crystal/gemstone under your pillow at night whilst you are asleep; thus, allowing the energies of the stone to gently penetrate your subtle body throughout the course of the night.

The healing - and therapeutic - power of crystals and gemstones has even reached boardroom level!

In some natural health exhibitions, for example, I have sold some large Amethyst clusters to Managing Directors, Sales Directors etc. who have acquired these big clusters to place on their office desks - or within their boardroom!

Amethyst or Quartz crystal clusters are now the 'in' executive toy.

Certain crystals and gemstones can help you to develop your spiritual abilities and gifts. Use an Amethyst for developing your intuitive awareness; a Lapis Lazuli for acquiring wisdom and truth; a Moonstone for obtaining humanitarian love and sensitivity.

Use your crystals and gemstones wisely in the pursuit of all your ambitions and needs.

Be aware, however, that your crystals and gemstones can never become miracle workers. They need your loving care and attention, your mental attunement with their unique healing properties and energies, before they are able to truly help you!

If you look within the pages of any Book about Crystals and Gemstones you will see many thousands of crystals and gemstones listed, describing their geological characteristics.

Obviously, however, it would be totally impractical for any crystal healer or Crystal Reiki Therapist to include every single crystal and gemstone in their crystal collection!

We have therefore carefully selected a relatively small number of crystals and gemstones to include in this book and which we hope you will find very helpful when deciding which crystals and/or gemstones to use for the benefit of your patients/clients.

Remember when using any of the crystals/gemstones in the following list, use your reiki energies/symbols as well as your crystal healing energies to charge the crystals/gemstones with all your powerful healing energies to amplify the energies already present within the crystal/gemstone.

In all the workshops, courses, and seminars it is good to teach all students to use their intuition when choosing which crystals/gemstones to use and which crystal healing or crystal reiki configuration technique to use in their healing sessions.

Crystal Healing/Crystal Reiki should *never* be robotic. Every client/patient is unique; each one needs an individual healing session, even if they may have a similar health challenge to another client/patient.

****

Abalone: A stone for strengthening the muscular tissue, especially around the heart. Very good in the treatment of spinal degenerative diseases and healing skeletal structure. Beneficial in relaxing the nervous system, brings feelings of relaxation and wellbeing. Encourages peace and tranquillity. Good for any emotional issues and emotional and spiritual growth

Agate: Semi-precious stone, said to improve natural vitality and energy and to increase the self-confidence of the wearer. Agate stabilises and strengthens the mind and body, aids general healing, reduces fever, hardens tender gums, gives courage and banishes fear. Helps to develop powers of eloquence. Stone of good health and fortune.

Fire Agate is believed to be especially beneficial to athletes and those taking any kind of examination or test, or anyone who has to call upon sudden bursts of mental or physical energy. Increases stamina, energy and circulation. Helps one come fully into the body in life force, creativity, expression. Activates and heightens the senses, brings pleasure and positivity.

Ajoite: Calming and blancing. Helps to soothe the nervous system and provide a more balanced and serene energy. Brings clarity and focus whilst remaining in a centred, peaceful state. Can aid in calming and balancing ADHD symptoms of either hyperactive or inattentive. Many report the feeling of this crystal having somewhat an angelic energy. Very good all round balancer and energetic body strengthener for all the energy systems of the body and the auric, biomagnetic and polyhedral fields.

Albite: Strengthens the lungs, circulatory system, spleen and thymus. Brings mental clarity and improves cognitive function. Good for issues of the brain and can improve memory. Relieves stress.

Alexandrite: Helps the nervous system, spleen, pancreas, and testicles. May be used to amplify colour therapy. Aids resilience, good for grief and matters of the heart. Good in times of change or emotional work, aids perception and understanding.

Amazonite: Helps Thyroid and Adrenal glands. Generally used to help soothe the nervous system and to give relief to those suffering from emotional disturbances and bring emotional harmony. Also helps with cell metabolism and regeneration. Useful when trying to express oneself more clearly after repression. Regulates and improves thinking abilities linked to one's integrity and values.

Amber: Not really a stone, but the yellow-brown fossilised resin of trees. Used to best effect by those suffering from tooth and gum problems, teething babies, throat infections, bronchial disorders or those prone to asthma or convulsions.

Also useful for rheumatism, intestinal disorders, earache, bladder trouble, nerves or bone-marrow deficiencies. Calming. Absorbs negative energy and helps the body to heal itself. Used for making and breaking spells. Helps lift depression and suicidal tendencies.

Amethyst: A purple-coloured Quartz used as a semi-precious stone, the Amethyst is known as a spiritual stone and is used for general healing and meditation.

It is said that sleeping with a piece of Amethyst beneath one's pillow promotes intuitive dreams and inspired thought. Many healers consider it useful for the relief of insomnia and to bring solace in times of grief. Amethyst clears, purifies and helps with addictions, stress or tension.

It also protects against blood disease, the toxic effects of substance use, acne, neuralgia, and fits. Soothes and calms the mind, raises the spirit, re-balances and increases intuitive awareness, protects from negative vibrations. Traditionally believed to protect from drunkenness.

Anhydrite: Strengthens the kidneys and ovaries. Good for alleviating stress and bringing balance to the systematic whole. Reduces inflammation and promotes healing of the skin. Promotes peace, relaxation and emotional balance.

Apache Tear: Used in 'grounding' one's energies; also helps soul reflection. Energy Protection. Can be used to work through feelings of grief or repressed emotions. Cleanses and purifies the auric field. Brings self strength and reliance.

Apatite: Strengthens muscle tissue, helps in coordinating basic motor responses. Helps those who suffer from stuttering and is also used in the treatment of hypertension, dizziness and vertigo. Stimulates the mind, enhances perception and brings clarity in deep thinking.

Aqua-Aura: Improves the heart, lungs, throat, and thymus. Good for those suffering from emotional trauma. Aids release of inner emotional tension and stress from deep within the body, issues of communication and connection. Helps meditation. Brings tranquillity and peace. Balances the mental and physical body,

Aquamarine: A bluish-green transparent beryl, the Aquamarine is believed to be most useful when dealing with problems of the eyes, liver, throat, stomach, nerves, and glands. Soothes skin disorders. Relieves toothache, improves sight. Aids healing inflammatory diseases. Preserves innocence. Quickens intellect, increases self-knowledge.

It is also reputed to promote clear, calm and logical thinking and for that reason is often carried as a 'good luck' charm by those taking examinations or being interviewed for a job.

Atacamite: Strengthens the genitals, thyroid, thymus gland and the nervous system. Used in the treatment of venereal diseases, including herpes. Aids communication and expression. A great meditational stone for relieving stress and for strengthening connection to self and spirit.

Aventurine: Said to be useful in relieving migraine and in soothing the eyes. A traditional method of using this stone is to make an elixir and bathe the eyes in the water the following day.

Aventurine water can also be useful for bathing irritations of the skin. Aventurine is a soother and helps relax one for a better night's sleep. It also relieves tension and shock.

Improves vitality, equalises blood pressure. Can help regulate the heart and circulatory system. Encourages creativity, gives the wearer courage, independence, and serenity.

Auralite: General energetic balancer for all energetic systems and can function at a cellular level for regeneration and rejuvenation. Great mediational tool for advanced awareness. Can aid in easing anxiety and depression and easing chronic issues of the body and mind.

Azurite: A natural blue copper carbonate, said to be an aid to psychic development, azurite is a very powerful stone, especially when placed on the third eye. It aids meditation and can penetrate your deepest subconscious fears. Physically it can help relieve tension headaches, migraines, Tinnitus and vertigo. It can also be used to relieve arthritis, joint disabilities and reduce hip and joint pain.

Beryl: Helps with heart problems, liver trouble, mouth, stomach and throat infections. Improves intellect, strengthens willpower, guards against lack of focus, failing senses and mental disorders. Beryl's prove to be good for overall health and wellbeing.

Also see: Aquamarine, Emerald, Morganite.

Bloodstone: A deep-green precious stone flecked with red, bloodstone is believed to help overcome depression and melancholia, especially when worn by the sufferer. It is also said to help those who suffer from psychosomatic illness and pains which have an emotional rather than a physical cause. Bloodstone purifies the blood and detoxifies the organs, particularly the liver, kidneys and spleen. It helps to allow light into the body. Provides vitality, strengthens idealism and the will to do good. Increases one's talent, stimulates the kundalini and balances all of the chakras.

Blue-lace Agate: Blue-lace agate is a very calming stone helpful for the throat chakra and freely expressing and remaining comfortable in oneself. Calms an overactive mind and racing thoughts. Good for thyroid and thymus glands. Eases inflammation, infections and fevers. Provides calming and soothing energy which can alleviate worry and anxiety.

Blue Quartz: Helps improve heart, lungs, throat and thymus. Good for people suffering from emotional trauma. Aids the release of inner emotional tension from deep within the body. Helps calm and relax the nervous system and is beneficial for meditation.

Boji Stone: Has general healing qualities and assists tissue regeneration. Strengthens all the chakras and meridians.

Boji stones can transfer energy from the etheric to the physical body. It will clean, recharge and fill with positive energy. Mends all of the voids or holes in the aura and the auric field.

In Atlantis, Boji stone energy was used for refining energy within each cell by placing a Boji stone on each chakra. When one or two Boji stones are set on the right polarity of the body, all pain may be removed within minutes.

Bornite: Bornite is one of the strongest healing stones in the mineral kingdom. It has the ability to align every chakra when applied to a given chakra. The energy within Bornite creates a circular, clockwise motion. Even though it is placed on one chakra, it will affect the other six.

It can cause a transformation that removes negative energy and replaces it with a strong, beneficial, positive energy. It possesses the unique property of energising not only the area on which it is placed, but all affects all of the surrounding area as well. Bornite is a very powerful mineral.

Calcite (yellow/gold): Carries the golden healing ray. Gives comfort, stimulation, helps lift depression. Good for most inactivity and lethargy, aids health and vitality. Aids metabolism and circulation

Calcite (green): Helps the kidneys, spleen and pancreas. Removes toxins from the body and alleviates mental fear. Aids mental clarity, soothes anxiety, calms turbulent energies. Expands awareness, aids intuition, links parallel realities. Good when undertaking mental change.

Calcite (orange/red): Helps the gallbladder, improves physical energy and expands awareness. Brings vitality and energy to the energetic systems. Good for the reproductive organs and regulating hormones.

Calcite (optical): Improves eyesight. Stimulates energy flow throughout the body and aura. Brings spiritual understanding into challenging circumstances and situations. Helps when doing regression for accessing and releasing the past. Also aids in creation, giving clear thought, removing stagnation.

Carnelian: Semi-precious stone, a reddish variety of Chalcedony.

Useful for understanding one's rhythms and cycles and it is said that if worn in a pouch around the neck by women during menstruation Carnelian will help to ease stomach cramps.

Strengthens voice. Helps rheumatism and arthritis, depression, neuralgia. Aids the sense of touch. Used for infertility and impotence. Alleviates blood poisoning, fever, infection and nose bleeds. Helps in the treatment of sores, spasms and wounds.

Protects from negative energy, elevates the spirit, grounds energies thus assisting concentration by clearing the mind and focusing one's thoughts. Helps daydreamers and those who are absent-minded. Provides vigour and energy.

Celestite: Helps to ease tension, opens and clears the mind and develops mental awareness. Cools the overactive mind, helps to relax muscles. Elevates consciousness. Promotes peaceful co-existence and harmonious interaction with other aspects of creation.

Chalcedony: Improves bone-marrow, spleen, red corpuscles and heart tissue. Stimulates optimism and enhances spiritual and artistic creativity. Good for calming anger, frustration and unease and strengthening the ability to respond and strengthen in mental, emotional, vocal and other expressive ways.

Chalcopyrite (Peacock Ore): Grounds and stabilises. Helps cheer those with constant worries and bring positivity and strength. Also improves prosperity consciousness. Removes energy blockages, stagnation and sluggishness. Balances the chi energy within the body and strengthens the systems as a whole. Can also aid in eliminating toxins.

Charoite: Dissolves fear including the fear of fear itself! Will help the fear rise to the surface so that it may be faced and dealt with. Good mental, emotional and spiritual healer. Helps aid transformations through growth. Good for fluid regulation within the body. Strengthens brain and thought process. Clears negativity, aids in emotional and energetic boundaries

Chrysocolla: Regulates thyroid and adrenals. Aids inflammation, issues and infections of the throat. Rids emotional congestion, ulcer or stomach problems. Brings balance, calm, inner peace and contentment. Cleanses all negativity. Aids in the release of stress, tension and anxiety. Dispels fear, judgement, criticism and negative thinking.

Chrysolite: An iron magnesium silicate. Strengthens the appendix. Alleviates general toxaemia and viral conditions. Eliminates toxins, strengthens the liver and gallbladder and can aid digestion. Chrysolite is good for overall health and gener al wellbeing.

Chrysoprase: Improves prostate gland, testicles, fallopian tubes and ovaries. Increases fertility. Aids in healing, regeneration and recuperation from all degenerative diseases. Chrysoprase balances symptoms that occur due the emotional messaging to the body, it will aid in allowing the brain and body a more harmonious feedback, alleviating symptoms of emotional and physical stress,restlessness, anxiety and other physical responses.

Citrine: Yellow variety of Quartz. Claims to give a sense of direction to those who feel they have lost their path in life.

Helps to control the emotions and works with relationships and self-knowledge. Attracts self-worth, gives confidence, dissolves emotional blocks, and induces dreams. Also said to be beneficial to people suffering from poor circulation. Strengthens the immune system, aids tissue regeneration.

Eases toxic conditions particularly in the endocrine and digestive systems. Helps with diabetes and depression. Activates mental powers and clarifies thought.

Improves self-image bringing confidence into relationships and environment, improving the quality of one's life, sometimes bringing prosperity. Reduces harmful effects of electrical products.

Conichalcite: A form of green Chlorite. Aids in detoxification and improved function of the kidneys and bladder. Can aid the body's recovery from ailments and surgery. Cheering stone, easing anxiety and stress, also aids in strength and courage in times of sorrow or change. helpful with symbolic re-birth, helps strengthen new resolutions.

Coral: Hard substance formed of skeletons of various marine polyps. Said to promote general physical and mental wellbeing and to help in particular those suffering from anaemia, bladder conditions, colic and whooping cough. In many parts of the world, it is believed that coral can be used to ward off evil thoughts sent by well-wishers.

Crocoite: Stimulates general health and vitality. Helpful for strengthening the immune system and the endocrine system. Helpful to those who have become regressed by perceived limitations or emotional hardship. Aids one in higher thinking and understanding for enlightenment.

Danburite: When worn or carried or used in a layout this stone helps one to maintain a strong sense of self identity while still preserving the knowledge of themselves as part of a greater whole. Helps you to acknowledge your personal growth on your path of self-realisation. Gives clarity and harmony of thought and mind.

Diamond: Master healer. Stimulates and balances all of the energy centres and surrounds of the physical body. Great tool to be used directly on the body. An extremely powerful stone used for the removal of physical blockages and all emotional negativities as it can balance the brain functions.

Dioptase: An emerald, green silicate of copper. A general healer which relieves mental stress. Promotes abundance, relaxation, love, and emotional expressiveness. Heals the parts emotionally abandoned while experiencing heartache. Good for those who, through loss, fear to love again, helps heal the heart and helps one to be able to trust again.

Dolomite: Used to help those who lack resourcefulness and who have an acute fear of personal failure. It lends a calming and peaceful energy for steady momentum forward in emotional matters. Aid in soothing the nervous system and bringing stable support for the body to function optimally as a whole.

Emerald: Bright green precious stone that improves intellect and memory. Helps tired eyes and insomnia. Improves eloquence. Good for strengthening the heart and heart function. Aids in strengthening from heart problems and surgery. Gives higher consciousness and has been known to help those see into the future. Known to bring luck and grant success in business. Acts as an emotional healer and stabiliser. Said to help release emotionally based trauma. Opens the heart to love, peace and deep healing.

Fluorite: Helps bring the spiritual into the material and quickens enlightenment. Helps heal holes in one's aura where energy is drained. Grounds, balances, and focuses one's energies. Absorbs and alters negative and other energies.

Opens the chakras. Aids physical and mental healing. Strengthens bone tissue, especially tooth enamel. Relieves dental disease, pneumonia, viral inflammation, sinus problems and ear issues. Brings clarity of mind, good for study, concentration and focus.

Galena: Strengthens lungs, thyroid, and the nervous system. Protects against depression and skin diseases. Promotes self-confidence, pride and success. Improves imagination.

Garnet: Most frequently used as a general tonic for the whole system - physical, mental, and emotional. It is regenerative and revitalising, strengthens the blood and helps with anaemia and circulatory problems.

Protects against infection, depression, and skin diseases. Brings into consciousness the physical powers and is particularly recommended for those who need to improve their self-respect and self-confidence and to increase courage when dealing with changes.

Improves imagination. Assists in dream work and in past life recall. Increases determination, energy, and courage. Attracts love, promotes bonding.

Gem Silica (Chrysoprase): Apple green variety of chalcedony. Reveals will-power and is useful for dealing with depression and loss of incentive.

Feminine stone, ideal for menstrual pain and premenstrual tension. Helps after miscarriage, abortions, hysterectomies. Helps with birthing if held, worn or meditated upon during labour.

Cools fever, heals burns, calms nerves, helps thyroid imbalance, voice problems, neck and shoulder strain. Develops patience, kindness, tolerance, compassion, humility. Gives peace and serenity, emotional balance, eases sorrow and anger. Good for men who, traditionally, find it difficult to express their feelings or emotions.

Excellent stone for meditation and can assist the development of clairvoyance.

Grossuralite: Used in the treatment of people who fear emotional hostility from everyone surrounding them. Brings calm communication and expression. Anti-inflammatory, good for Arthritis, Rheumatoid and autoimmune conditions.

Hematite: A natural ferric oxide, hematite improves all blood disorders. Reduces stressful effects of air travel, combats insomnia. Enhances astral projection, promotes balance, focus, convergence and concentration of energy. Said to increase courage. Also claimed to strengthen the heart and is good for reducing a rapid pulse.

Herderite: This stone stimulates the pancreas and spleen and helps to restore the balance in erratic emotional behaviour.

Herkimer Diamond: Releases stress and tension throughout the body, aids in any physical healing, increases, amplifies the power of other crystals by being used to close the circuit, particularly effective with Boji stones.

Balances physical, mental, emotional and energetic fields, clearing blockages and heightening consciousness. Can provide some pain relief when applied on that part of the body.

Howlite (magnetite): Aids digestive system, abdomen and upper intestinal tract. Soothes the nervous system. Eases anxiety, depression, frustration, stress, worry and gives a clarity and calm to racing thoughts

Strengthens astral body. Opens mind to new ideas, intellectually stimulating, links left and right hemispheres of the brain facilitating communication between logic and emotion. Promotes powers of analysis and creativity, psychic development, memory, channelling activities, strength of will.

Iolite: calms mind, emotions, clears thought process and strengthens intuition. Eliminates toxins and fat deposits. Helps headaches and migraines. Heals old wounds, strengthens connection to self and spirit.

Ivory: Protects the physical body from injury. Balances masculine and feminine sides. Strengthens immune system.

Jacinth: Promotes spiritual sight and understanding. Used in childbirth. Helps in the treatment of insomnia.

Jade: A pale green gemstone said to help in relieving kidney complaints, bladder trouble and eye problems.

Yellow jade is believed to aid poor digestion. When worn as a piece of jewellery, jade is thought to provide protection from one's enemies and can be used for protection on long journeys.

Also used to attract good luck, for wisdom, for long life and a peaceful death. Helps to control dream content. In ancient China and Egypt it was widely used as a talisman to attract good fortune, friendship and loyalty.

Jasper: Coloured impure form of natural silica said to be both invigorating and stabilising, bringing stillness to a troubled mind. Generates an even rhythmic pulse and is also said to improve the sense of smell and to overcome depression.

Red jasper is known to contain iron oxide which is used medically to control excessive bleeding. It is claimed, therefore, that it can be useful in overcoming disorders of the blood. Also used for digestion and stomach problems, biliousness and bladder trouble. Protects from witchcraft, soothes the nerves.

Jet: A very hard lustrous form of natural carbon. Prevents deep depression, quietens fears. Protects from violence and illness. Aids grieving. Also used in healing to control and ease migraine and pain behind the eyes.

Kunzite: Alleviates anaemia, improves general tissue rejuvenation. Supports the nervous system and parasympathetic nervous system, Creates balance between heart and mind, clears emotional blockages. In meditation it can balance negative emotional and troubled mental states. Brings calm and acceptance of oneself.

Kyanite: Used in meridian points to stimulate flow of energy, or on chakra centres to clear blockages. Recalls past lives when placed on the third eye. Augments channelling, altered states, vivid dreams, clear visualisation, loyalty, honour and serenity.

Kyanite blades can make incisions in the auric field. Can also cut through layers of mental misconceptions and create new lines of energy for new thought.

Labradorite: A stone of transformation and for transition. Helps with meditation and focus. A good all round balancer physically and mentally. Helps one to hone their intuition and creativity, inspiring movement and personal growth. Physically it can be useful to aid the digestive system and regulate metabolism and the nervous system.

Labradorite is also known as the stone of Odin and is said to give the user a sense of connection to 'magic' and the mystery of the greater whole and being.

It is commonly gifted to friends that live at a distance as a source of connection and for continued communication. It can not only help with telepathic communication but aids dreams and dream recall, helping one to be more in tune with their subconscious and psyche.

Lapis Lazuli: A brilliant blue mineral, the lapis lazuli was called the Stone of Heaven by the ancient Egyptians and is thought by many to be the stone upon which were carved the laws given to Moses.

It is said to prevent fits and epilepsy and to improve eyesight. Helps heart and spleen, protects against strokes, helps lift depression. Also helps with the acquisition of wisdom and truth. A symbol of power and a mental and spiritual cleanser. Assists psychic development and mental stability. Gives hope and self-awareness and helps one face one's shadow self. The stone of friendship. Helps cut through superficialities to find inner truth. Aura cleanser.

Larimar: Soothes sore throats and tonsillitis. Helps express new ideas. Brings harmony between heart and mind. Good for schizophrenia, Transmutes anger, greed, frustration to peace; calms excess energies by rebalancing. Cleanses, soothes and Eases Inflammation.

Lazulite: Improves and stimulates the pineal glands and liver. Boosts immune system and endocrine glands. Balances energy, gives relief from worry or tension. Helps with relaxation and balance of an overactive mind. Helpful for headaches and migraines. Said to aid one in identifying and releasing emotional patterns.

Lazurite: Stimulates visions and amplifies thought-form. Very good for balancing the brain and mental clarity, also used for tissue rejuvenation, boosting immunity and giving vitality and strength.

Lazurite can also assist in dreams, dream recall and astral projection. This stone finds a balance between earth and higher energies - harmony with nature and expansion to the divine. It allows one to take a step back and see the bigger picture. It works on a level of balanced inner and outer reflection assisting personal growth.

Lepidolite: Unifies mind and heart, heals whatever inhibits this merging. Used in the treatment of schizophrenia. Calms the mind, aids in sleep, meditation and relaxation. Reduces stress and depression. Benefits emotions and hormones and emotional and mental imbalances.

Lepidolite with Rubellite: Good for introverted, shy people who are unable to express love in external ways. Supports those with social anxiety or nervous disposition. Eases restlessness and balances energy flow.

Rubellite supports by giving courage, strength and vitality. Physically it can benefit the bloodstream, veins and blood circulation.

The combination of Lepidolite and Rubellite gives a higher sense of self and purpose, alleviating stress and redirecting energy in a healthy positive manner. It allows for a calm and cleansed heart space where one can find love, intuition and trust in oneself.

Sugilite: Restores balance to pineal, pituitary and left and right brain hemispheres. Helps ease headaches, epilepsy, dyslexia, physical coordination, visual problems, spiritual problems. Sugilite is a great stone to work with in times of upheaval, struggle or unhappiness. It promotes calm serenity and optimism going forward, supporting one in not losing their peace. Acts as a stabiliser for Autism, A.D.H.D, and anyone who feels highly sensitive.

Magnetite: Stimulates the endocrine system. Improves blood circulation. Helps in meditation. You can place Magnetite on an area or wound to increase blood and lymph flow to facilitate healing. Helps ground and recuperate from energetic burnout and fatigue. Can help with mood swings and keeping the emotions steady.

Malachite: A green copper carbonate, Malachite contains copper and is claimed to be helpful in the treatment of arthritis and rheumatism. Supports formation of healthy red blood cells and haemoglobin and can also help regulate menstruation. Reduces inflammation and can relieve physical pain when placed on the body. Used also in the treatment of asthma and the respiratory system. Helps toothache. Improves eyesight.

Raises one's spirits and increases hope, health and happiness. Attracts physical and material benefits and brings prosperity as one takes action. Assists wise rule and helps remove mental blockages hindering spiritual growth. Relieves any congestion in the body and helps with confusion, a lack of purpose and insecurity.

Marcasite: Gentle physical strengthener and vitality giver. Makes one feel more able to cope with any problems and difficulties. Good for issues with the skin and mucous membranes.

Mimetite: Helps communication; grounds and balances emotions. Nourishing and rejuvenating, good for boosting concentration and optimism, provides peace and serenity to those who feel vulnerable or emotionally fragile.

Moldavite: Tektite associated with high vibrational healing and extraterrestrial connection.

Powerful cleansing and clearing of energy blockages. Allows energy and current flow through the body. Ultimate high consciousness access and ascension stone. Aids profound mediations, subconscious thoughts and lucid dreams.

Eases epilepsy, brain imbalances and malfunctions and autism, particularly if brought on by excessive sensitivity.

Assists conscious communication with star-seed sources and is a healing balm for the deep longing of many people to 'go home'. Moldavite also helps one to understand one's true purpose in life. A stone for profound self and life transformation!

Rainbow Moonstone: Moonstone is an opalescent feldspar claimed to promote long life and happiness and said to attract friendship and loyalty towards the wearer.

Acts as a mediator between mind and emotions and allows peace of mind and accessibility to one's inner self. Helps soothe and balance emotions. Useful for healing heavy heart emotions and grief. Physically it is often used to reduce excess fluid in the body and to reduce any attendant swelling. Used for women suffering from premenstrual tension. Gives inspiration, encourages personal attachments. Helps obtain humanitarian love, romance, and sensitivity.

Morganite: Strengthens the larynx, lungs, thyroid and nervous system and can aid in endurance and stamina. Calms the mind. Emotionally, Morganite is used for strengthening matters of the heart, Can bring feelings of peace and acceptance. Allows one to be receptive to emotions, vulnerability and to feel protected in matters of heart space, boundaries and love itself.

Morion Crystal: A Smokey Quartz crystal so dark it seems black instead of the more usual brown. Very good for grounding, stability and protection. Soothes, balances and regulates the system as a whole.

Morion Smokey makes a very good gridding crystal on or around the body and place that is required to have more energetic balance and protection. It is especially helpful for auric leaks and balancing the energy and sealing it.

Moss-Agate: Brings balance, stability and grounding. Cleanses the emotional body and calm temperament, helps to release anger and frustration. Strengthens the physical and etheric body. Enhances senses and perception, good for concentration and memory. Can help one connect to the earth and nature, giving peaceful, harmonious energy.

Anti inflammatory, helps support the lymphatic system and eliminate toxins. A great stone to have to help fight infections, inflammation and for aiding quick recovery after illness.

Can also be used on skin to help calm skin issues, rejuvenate skin and influence correct Ph.

Obsidian Snowflake: A grounding stone that makes the user face up to responsibility. Helps one to find and utilise the strength within. Dedicated to change, metamorphosis, purification, fulfilment, inner growth and introspection. Deflects negative energy. Removes blockages and cleanses the energy field.

Onyx: A variety of agate, the onyx is reputed to improve concentration and devotion which is perhaps why it is frequently found in rosaries.

Helps hearing problems, heart trouble and ulcers. Can give inner strength and introspection for balance, self mastery. Calm nerves and anxiety, bringing balance and clear mental channel for consistent forward movement, even in trying times.

Opal: Helps lung conditions, increases assimilation of protein. Assists the control of one's temper and calms the nerves. Helps calm and clarify the emotional body bringing focus and nurturing.

Aids the development of psychic ability. Sometimes considered an unlucky stone, perhaps because it causes one's thoughts, good or bad, to rebound.

Above all, it is a stone of emotions and love, but if the lover is false its influence is reversed, and the opal proves a sorry stone for faithless lovers.

Pearl: The only gem born from a conscious, nurturing process. Their origin is the result of a living being choosing to self nurture. Shamans and healers throughout the ages have promoted this stone for relaxation, introspection and self love and healing.

Physically it has been known to have helped lung disorders such as asthma, bronchitis and emphysema and tuberculosis. Pearl promotes antibodies and fights infection, reduces fever and is useful for allergies. When in powder form it can help inflammation and healing of the skin.

Peridot: Peridot, as well as being recommended as a cure for insomnia, is said to aid the digestion and placate the nervous system.

Improves bruised eyes. Can cleanse and heal hurt feelings, helps mend damaged relationships. Develops inner vision, the stone of the seer. Counteracts negativity and opens the mind. Acts like a tonic, heals the physical body and can be useful in reducing fever. Also used in treating emotional states such as anger and jealousy.

Petrified Wood: Restores physical energy. Helps hip and back problems. Builds strength and stability. Aids past-life recall and connection to ancestors. Grounding and aids sleep disorders and brings a gentle nurturing energy and inner peace.

Picasso Marble (Picasso Jasper): Picasso Marble (or Picasso Stone) has strong metaphysical qualities of grounding and calming. It also promotes weight loss and assists in the development of creativity, as well as engendering strength and self-discipline.

Pietersite (Tempest Stone): Pietersite, sometimes known as TheTempeststone, helps one see beyond the immediate to beauty in the all. Brings insight and intuition. It enhances courage, tenacity, and ability to maintain or create what is yours.

Spiritually and physically, Pietersite helps in working with angels, experiencing visions, and precognition, relating to feminine or goddess energy, as well as astral and dimensional travel. Emotionally Pietersite helps to relax, and release deep emotions in a calmer way. It helps overcome inattentiveness, indecision and uncertainty. Can improve cognitive function and memory.

Physically, Pietersite balances body fluids, improves nutrition, helps with gastrointestinal functions, and helps the endocrine glands, balances female hormones, alleviates PMS and menopause symptoms.

Pyrite: Believed to increase the oxygen supply in the blood and tissues, strengthens the circulatory and endocrine systems, purifies the body of infection and is said to be useful in clearing congested passages.

Brings stability, stamina, strength and courage for forward movement and healing. Pyrite stimulates and enhances energy, giving support, mental clarity and focus.

Quartz Crystal: A natural crystalline silica, the Quartz crystal attracts the powers of light and energy and is said to be a powerful general all encompassing healer and powerful dynamic working tool. It works on all levels - strengthening, clearing, cleansing and protecting.

Purifies the air and surrounding area or room. Protects against harmful electrical vibrations.

Assists the wearer to think intuitively. Amplifies and transmits subtle vibrations. The symbol of elemental wholeness, containing the four elements of creation. Assists the development and integration of one's entire being. Helps one to amplify, focus, direct, transmit and store energy.

It is used as an aid to opening the psychic centres, enabling meditation at a deeper level and the liberation of one's mind from the mundane and the trivial, is considered to be its greatest attribute. Quartz crystal releases the higher consciousness and develops mystical and spiritual gifts.

Rhodochrosite: Prevents mental breakdowns, balances physical and emotional traumas. Improves eyesight, kidney, pancreas and spleen. Inspires forgiveness, heals emotional scars, attracts love. Helps one face reality and new situations. Assists integration of physical, mental and emotional fields. Good for soft tissues and the reproductive system in women.

Rhodonite: Restores physical energy, especially following trauma or shock. Strengthens inner ear and improves sense of hearing. Aids vitamin absorption. Boosts the immune system and can aid in autoimmune conditions. Increases language skills and communication, raises self-esteem. Helps maintain a loving state in everyday life by bolstering one's resolve not to give in without having to be aggressive. Restores physical and emotional strength.

Rhyolite: Rejuvenates physical beauty. Helps increase self-expression and the ability to speak with greater clarity. Known as a stone of the heart and for transition. Rhyolite comes in many types, colours and names and you may also hear these forms labelled as 'Jasper'. They all have differences and can be used based on intuitive connection, colour, look or vibration.

Rock Crystal: Relieves diarrhoea, dizziness, haemorrhage, kidney troubles, spasms, vertigo. Helps ease pain anywhere.

Rose Quartz: Claimed to be one of the best stones to use in the treatment of migraines and headaches of all types. Calms emotions, helps suffering due to emotional trauma, heals wounds of neglect. Also said to stimulate the imagination and intellect and to open the heart to inner peace, self-love, self-recognition and self-acceptance.

A very healing stone for internal wounds, bitterness, and sorrows, it promotes forgiveness, love and friendship. Makes one more receptive to beauty, hastens recovery and gladdens the heart. Known as the love stone.

Ruby: A deep red transparent gemstone, a form of corundum. As well as aiding intuitive thinking, it raises levels of energy and divine creativity.

Often used to alleviate disorders of the blood, such as anaemia, poor circulation and menstrual problems. Also used in the treatment of rheumatism and arthritis. Improves fever, pain and spasms. Alleviates worries, lifts spirit, improves confidence, intuition, spiritual wisdom, energy and courage. Encourages self-nurturing in those with a poor self-image.

Rutilated Quartz: Rutilated Quartz is said to be of particular benefit to those who suffer from respiratory complaints such as asthma, bronchitis and Emphysema.Increases tissue regeneration.

Rebalances different levels of consciousness. Heightens awareness. Improves decisiveness, focus and clarity. Strengthens one's will and courage going forward with its harmonious yet supportive and vibrant energies. Helps one to feel joy and content in themselves and life.

Sapphire: Helps control of bleeding, insomnia, and nervousness. Can help with eye problems, headaches and sinus issues. A stone known for having a strong third eye and crown chakras, enhancing psychic abilities, visions and stimulating dreams. Strengthens one's resolve and security within themselves and their abilities. Stone of wisdom, friendship and love, it attracts good influences. Gives the wearer devotion, faith, imagination, and peace of mind.

Sardonyx: Stimulates self-control and protection. Aids bravery and motivation in times of upheaval and new direction. Regulates metabolism and intestinal health. Boosts immune system, blood circulation and alleviates symptoms of chronic illnesses.

Selenite: One of the most powerful healing stones, selenite calms and clears troubled minds and is useful in personal meditation and visualisation.

Stabilises the emotions, bringing them under control. Gives serene and calm energy aiding relaxation and the nervous system. Helps clarify one's innermost thoughts and to expand one's mental powers.

Used in past-life recall and in regression therapy. Can be used in any healing treatment for clearing energetic and etheric blockages but should only be used by a qualified crystal healing therapist who is able to handle and direct the powerful energies properly.

Serpentine: Serpentine, which is also called New Jade, is a beneficial and versatile stone. It replenishes one's physical and emotional energy in a soothing and gentle manner. It will help with emotional cleansing, psychic powers, and attract love and money. It is also used in the rise of the kundalini, facilitating the rise by opening a path that lessens discomfort.

Serpentine is an excellent stone for meditation. Physically serpentine eliminates parasite infections.

Smithsonite: Calms and clears, good to use in high-anxiety situations. Helps after nervous breakdowns, relaxes over-tense muscles, also good in childbirth. Neutralises red energies.

Smokey Quartz: Disperses negative patterns and vibrations and transmits a high quantity of light. Good luck talisman. Helps protect soldiers on active service. Grounding and connective, it is an all round good balancer and energy cleanser.

Improves abdomen, kidneys, pancreas and the sexual organs. Increases energy fertility. Encourages survival instincts. Stimulates and purifies energy centres. Grounds and stabilise energies, helps lift depression. Draws out and absorbs negative energies, replacing them with positive ones.

Snow Quartz: Strengthens immune system. A softer energy than clear quartz. Used in meditation, Snow Quartz gives serenity and powers of inner contemplation. Can be good for balancing energy thrown off by dysregulated emotions.

Sodalite: A good stone for over-sensitive and defensive people, improves courage and endurance. Balances and stills the mind and clears rigid thought patterns. Helps logical and rational thought, and intellect. Widens the perspective.

Blue Sodalite is reputed to assist in lowering blood pressure and balancing the metabolism. Aids sleep and relaxation.

Spinel: Attracts helping energies and reflects negative energies. Re-energises and revitalises in a strong yet gentle manner. Can aid in reducing tiredness and fatigue. Replenishes depleted energy stores and supports recovery from shock, illness and trauma. Gives strength and relieves resistance, allowing one to move forward in the right direction and energies with a sense of inspiration and acceptance.

Staurolite: Used to help people who suffer from over caution or doubt or are struggling to find decisive clarity and direction. Can also aid in decision making. Good stone for earth, nature and animal connection. Aids one in grounding and connecting to the earth's electromagnetic field. Physically it helps one find physical connection and grounding and balances the emotional body.

Sugilite: Great for a 'sensitive soul' or anyone feeling emotional disharmony and sensitivity. Powerful for spiritual or energy work, it acts as a protector from negative energy and influences but also enhances any spiritual self development, inner vision and energetic cleansing.

Physically this stone calms anxiety, the nervous system and can be helpful for sleep disorders and insomnia.

Thulite: A stone of the heart, physically and mentally. To help those who are resisting a condition or relationship which they regard as discouraging. Helps those with judgement of self and others to find acceptance, understanding, harmony, contentment and self love. Can help in raising happiness and joy and finding passion in life again, especially if someone feels hurt, shame or self loathing.

It can help one find the true cause of their emotional unhappiness or suffering and start to recognize and adapt to a more open response towards others and an enlightened perspective to one's own emotional growth and healing.

Can help bring more joy and positivity to anyone who feels more stress and quick emotional or energy changes.

Tiger's Eye: Claimed to counteract feelings of hypochondria and the onset of psychosomatic illness. Also gives a feeling of self-confidence.

Especially good for clear thinking and for seeing a problem objectively when confused or emotionally affected. Releases tension and develops will-power.

Good for asthma. Helps one to gain insight into one's own faults. Protects from negative energies. Attracts good luck.

Topaz (yellow): A yellowish transparent mineral, topaz helps to overcome stress and soothes nerves thereby helping one to achieve a deeper sleep. Also good for colds and flu. Strengthens blood vessels, improves blood circulation, varicose veins, sense of taste. Good for liver trouble. Improves the intellect, develops psychic abilities, calms both mind and body.

Topaz (Blue): A calming stone. Good for throat disorders. Inspires leadership ability, psychic insight, spiritual and artistic growth. Helps with clarity and concentration and communication of any kind. Very calming and relaxing stone, good for personal insight, meditation and relieving anxiety and upset.

(White): Believed to enhance mental ability, increase wisdom and soothe anger. A stone to help clarity and intention. Aligns the mind with the body for practical matters. Said to help with vision of the mind and eyes.

(Golden): Gives grounded, gentle energy. Good for supporting the kidneys and urinary system. Keeps the energetic body balanced as a whole and soothes the nervous system.

Tourmaline (general): Prevents lymphatic disease. Balances, protects, calms, gives self-confidence and cheerfulness. Attracts inspiration, good-will and friendship. Protects the wearer against misfortune and anaemia. Grounds high-frequency energies into the physicality. Useful for meditation.

Tourmaline (black or green): Strengthens nervous system, regulates blood pressure. Deflects and protects negative energy, attracts prosperity. Gives stability and strength. Great for protecting healers and holistic workers from physically feeling pain from a client.

Tourmaline (blue): Helps with all throat problems, thyroid, speech impediments. Promotes clear verbal expression, dissolves mental friction and emotional constriction.

Tourmaline carries a high electrical charge and if rubbed briskly one end becomes positive and the other negative. The resulting energy can be directed wherever peaceful energy is required.

Tourmaline (watermelon/pink): Heart balancer. Promotes understanding of self and emotions. Complete heart and emotional cleanser and healer, bringing calm and strength. Good for those with C.P.T.S.D and P.T.S.D heart break, grief. Promotes emotional regulation and wellbeing.

Turquoise: A bluish green precious stone, turquoise helps the ability to express oneself and verbalise freely. It is good for laryngitis and nervousness in speech.

It is said that turquoise will grow pale on a sickly person and recover its colour when returned to a healthy person. Can strengthen entire anatomy and helps improve all diseases. It is a good all round balancer and healer for mind and body.

Shields the wearer from harmful influences, attracts friendship. Used in meditation and also for the development of intuition. Brings wisdom and also reminds us of both our spiritual nature and our earthly inheritance and its beauty.

Unakite: Helps balance and gives stability. A grounding stone. Earthing and revitalising, it grounds whilst detoxing. Good for issues with the intestines and gastrointestinal tract. Can bring a sense of peace and patience.

Vanadinite: Helps with throat problems and communication. Excellent for anyone with physical jobs or athleticism to aid in stamina, vitality and energy. Said to aid fatigue and boost energy.

Vanadinite is a stone that can balance the physicality of the body with the mental power and workings of the mind, making it a powerful stone for earthly balance whilst providing mental clarity.

Vivianite: Symbol of rebirth burns away old ways of looking at things and gives one a new perspective on life. Helps clear vision at all levels. Brings deep peace and calm to the mind and heart space. A good emotional healer from trauma and fear. Aids in balancing the physical and emotional energies in the body and can aid the nervous system.

Zircon: General healer for balancing the mind and body, the inner and outer. Good for stimulating energies and energy flow of the chakras. Helps liver complaints, assists the bodily stress of childbirth, can relieve insomnia due to aiding in stress and providing calm consciousness.. Promotes spiritual sight and understanding.

Zoisite: Strengthens the male genitals and the female cervix. Helps to increase fertility.

Balances the heart energy and strengthens the connection between the heart and the head, making it a good ally for overall health and wellbeing when used intuitively for change and growth. Instills passion and action whilst also keeping one grounded and focused with intent.

NOTE: This list is in no way extensive and we also urge you to note your own findings with the crystals and the work you may undertake with them, whether they match up with the findings above or if they differ. Crystals can act like prescriptions and can affect people differently and work for people differently on many levels. Have fun with your findings and extending your knowledge!

Chapter 5: Crystal Reiki Reflexology

To do Crystal Reiki Reflexology, or foot massage treatment, select a quartz crystal which has a good polished, smooth single-terminated point.

Then ask your client to remove either their socks or their tights.

Crystal Reiki Reflexology treatments may either be done with the client lying on a massage couch, or sitting comfortably in a chair. When using the latter method, you will need to sit on a stool so that you can place your client's feet upon your lap.

Whether you choose to use a massage couch, or a chair for your treatment, you should also place several quartz crystals around the area where your crystal reiki reflexology client is either lying or sitting. The number of quartz crystals you need can be arrived at intuitively.

To give your client both reiki and reflexology in the same treatment session you need first to give them reiki healing in the way you would normally do and, of course, from this perspective, it doesn't much matter whether you client is lying on a massage couch or is sitting down on an ordinary dining room-type chair.

The principles of reflexology are that the feet consist of numerous reflex points; all of which relate to specific parts of the physical body.

An ordinary qualified reflexologist will use his/her hands to press into every one of these reflex points and when a health problem is diagnosed the client will often feel a sharp pain and the therapist will detect a small pea-like lump just under the surface of the skin.

To give you an idea of where all the main reflex points are in the feet, please study the chart below:

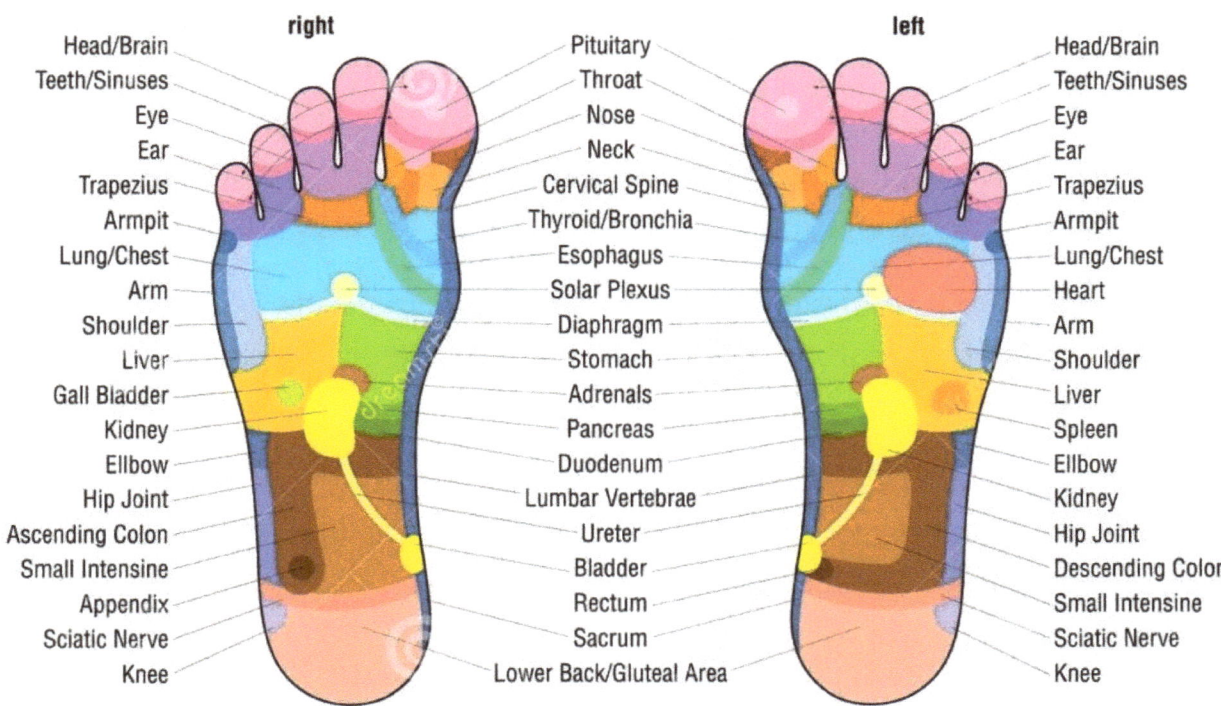

In crystal reiki reflexology, however, we do not need to be quite as precise as a reflexologist. First, naturally, we must program our healing quartz crystal to re-balance any imbalances which might be discovered in the client's body as the treatment proceeds.

Using the single-terminated end of the quartz crystal the crystal reiki healer will gently—and without pressing too deep into the skin—start to rotate the crystal in a clockwise direction on the skin of the feet.

Traditionally starting with the sole of the client's left foot, the crystal is moved slowly around to the sides, lightly touching the skin all the time, and then on to the upper part of the foot. All movements should be both slow and deliberate. Make sure that you cover all the surface of the foot. Then do the same with the right foot.

Whenever the crystal reiki healer obtains a reaction from the client, he or she should spend a few moments directing crystalline healing energy into the appropriate reflex point.

As the crystal reflexology treatment ends the crystal reiki therapist should take the quartz crystal and lightly run it over the entire surface of the foot, on the soles and on the upper part of both feet.

As a rough time-guide I would suggest that you spend around thirty minutes per foot but naturally this is completely flexible depending upon what you find and upon the needs of your client.

Once you have completed your crystal reiki reflexology treatment of both feet with your quartz crystal, then you should complete the treatment session by projecting some more reiki energies into your client before bringing them back into their normal consciousness.

Chapter 6: Crystal Reiki Massage

Crystal Reiki massage can be a beautiful and uplifting experience. It works on a deep esoteric level and not only does the physical body enjoy total relaxation, but all the inner emotional stresses and tensions are brought skillfully to the surface of the conscious mind and dissipated.

There are many and varied ways of using quartz crystals to enrich and enhance the massage experience.

Aromatherapy can also be used with crystals and gemstones.

Some therapists use polished Crystal palm stones for massaging the body, or Basalt for hot massage and they use Granite for cold therapy. Nowadays there are many Crystal wand tools, ranging from large to small, made for massage and reflexology, which are made out of Quartz crystal, Rose Quartz, Amethyst and Fluorite, to name a few. You can easily find them in a range of materials and prices on the market. While these massage tools may give an excellent crystal massage in a generic sense and allow for trigger pointing on the muscles, they can never really give your client much in the way of healing energies, especially in a short time, however you can program any crystals you use, Quartz is best. We prefer to use natural Quartz crystals which have no jagged edges.

Before you begin to use your Quartz crystal on your client, it is important that you first program it with the thought that the crystal vibrations and energies are going to merge with those of your client.

I always mentally attune myself to the crystal by asking that the crystal energies be absorbed into the skin of the client and that their body be totally re-energized, re-harmonized and rebalanced wherever any 'imbalances' are to be found.

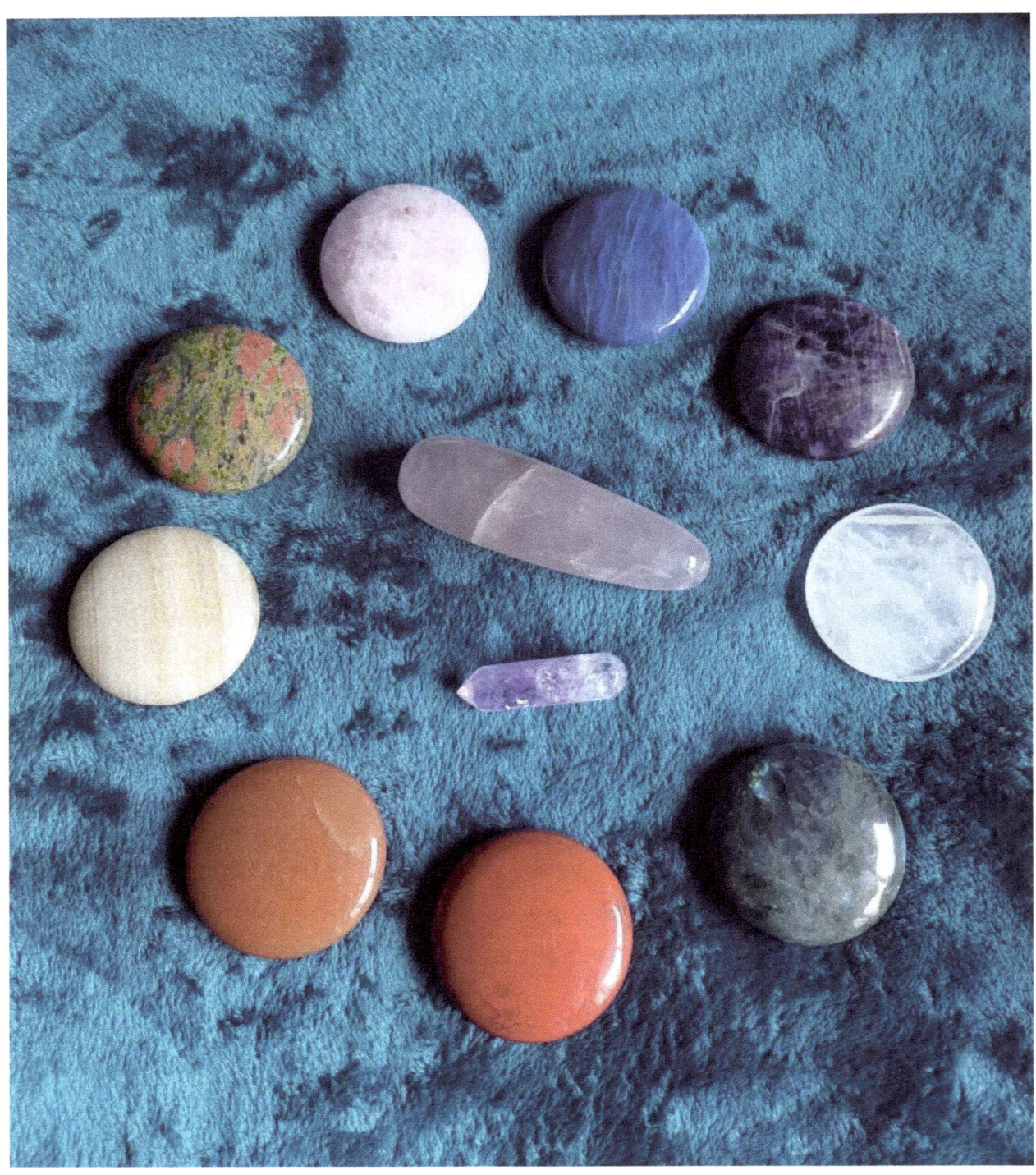

Once you have learnt and mastered ordinary crystal reiki healing techniques you can then move on to practising more advanced crystal reiki healing techniques.

Ketseuki Kokan Ho - Kekko Massage

Ketseuki Kokan Ho, was one of the main level 2 Reiki techniques taught by Dr. Hayasho. This technique is an effective treatment for a wide variety of problems, because it stimulates circulation, strengthens the flow of life force energy and promotes the release of toxins. According to Reiki tradition it is best used at the end of a Reiki treatment session.

To perform this technique, have the client lay face down on the healing table and perform the following steps:

1. Locate the indentations on either side of the neck and skull.
2. Place the thumb and index finger of one hand in the indentation, then visualise the power symbol there.
3. Place the index and middle finger of the other hand on either side of the clients spine at the base of the neck.
4. Swiftly run your fingers down along the spine to the sacrum, repeat this process 20 times.
5. Find the indentation on the sacrum and again, use the thumb and index finger, visualising the power symbol there.
6. Divide the upper part of the clients back into six areas, three on each side of the spine.
7. Brush across the small of the back, rubbing your hand side to side with slight pressure, repeat ten times.
8. Start at the hip and sweep your hand down along the outside of the leg to the ankle. Do both legs four times.
9. Start from the back of the thigh and sweep your hand down the back of the leg of the ankle. Do both legs four times.
10. Start from the inside of the lower thigh and sweep down from the ankle. Do both legs four times.

11. Pushing down on the base of the thigh just above the back of the knee, clasp the ankle with the other hand. Gently stretch the back of the knee. Do both legs.
12. Pat the back all over from the upper to the lower torso, do four times.
13. Pat down the legs in the same order as steps 8-10. Begin with the outside of the leg, then do the back of the leg, then the inside of the leg - alternating right and left legs.

Byosen scanning

A technique taught by Master Usui to all his students. This technique is a useful tool for identifying areas of energy blockages in the clients body and auric field.

To perform the Byosen scanning on your client, put your hands together in prayer position in front of your heart and ask for connection to your Reiki guides. Bring your hands up to your third eye (sixth chakra) and ask for guidance about where in the body or auric field of the client is experiencing problems.

If you are a Reiki Therapist/Healer and would like more information about Crystal Reiki Healing, please send an email to:
charleslightwalker@yahoo.com

For more information on Crystal Reflexology and Crystal healing email: mintakamermaid@gmail.com

Chapter 7: Star of David Crystal Reiki Configuration

The Star of David Crystal Reiki Configuration is a very important configuration in all your Crystal Reiki Treatments. The vibrational energies created by the crystals which go to make up this powerful Configuration assist in the amplification of all your crystal and reiki healing energies.

Your client should sit on the floor, in yoga fashion, or in a chair, holding a quartz crystal in the palm of their hand. Six quartz crystals should then be placed around them in the form of a six-pointed star.

The Star of David Crystal Reiki Configuration enables you to cover all aspects of your client's being and to correct the spiritual and physical energy flowing throughout their body. This particular configuration works very well to realign all emotional imbalances, helping to bring blockages to the surface of your client's conscious mind.

The Star of David Crystal Reiki Configuration can also be used very effectively with your client lying on their back. One quartz crystal should be placed at the head with the single-terminated end pointing away from the body. Two quartz crystals should be placed at the knees, pointing upwards.

When your client is within the Star of David Crystal Reiki Configuration you should take your personal healing control quartz crystal and energise the six configuration quartz crystals by directing your crystal over all of the crystals surrounding your client - do this several times.

Whilst you are actively energising the Star of David Crystal Reiki Configuration Crystals you should be programming the crystalline energies to rebalance all the imbalances within your clients physical and mental bodies.

And as your client lies very relaxed with their eyes closed inside the Configuration you may then intuitively project crystal and reiki healing energies into your client's body.

Your client should lie within this field of crystalline energy for between twenty to thirty minutes, although you may extend this period of time if you feel that is necessary.

(Charles) *Although, of course, it is not possible for any therapist to guarantee a cure, in my personal experience at least 80% of my clients, who receive healing from me within the Star of David Crystal Reiki Configuration feel much improved in their general health and, often, their health concerns become much lessened!*

8: Four Directions Crystal Reiki Layout

The four directions Crystal Reiki layout is mainly used for meditations and for 'charging' objects.

Place one crystal representing North (earth, wisdom, connectors), one representing South (fire, faith, protectors), one East (air, creativity, illuminators) and one West (water, sacred dreams, initiators). The single-terminated ends of each crystal should be pointing towards the centre.

Sit in the middle of this crystal reiki layout for fifteen to twenty minutes. You might like to hold a crystal cluster in your hands. Sit in the direction you feel compelled to face; many people like to sit facing east.

Visualise drawing down the appropriate Reiki Symbols into your physical body for whatever you need at this particular time.

If you decide to lie down in the Four Directions Crystal Reiki Layout, you should have your head facing north and your feet facing south. This aligns with the polarities of the earth.

Chapter 09: Crystal Reiki Relationship Configuration

If two people are in conflict with each other, perhaps through stress or misunderstanding, a pattern of double crystal reiki triangulations is strongly recommended.

This Crystal Reiki Relationship Configuration will help create an understanding between the two people in conflict and thus serve to establish a sound balance between the flows of their vibrations.

The two individuals should sit facing each other, approximately three feet apart, in the cross-legged, or if possible, lotus position.

They should each take two Quartz crystals and place them in a line behind themselves. Then they should place the third quartz crystal in a position that forms a triangle with the other two crystals, in front of them, with the single-terminated end facing the other person. The two should then meditate together and absorb the healing energies created by the double crystal reiki triangulation.

The effect you are creating is a symbolic one. You are taking the energies of the trinity of one and blending them with the energies of the trinity of the other. The results will be both healing and releasing and will create an understanding between the two in conflict.

Chapter 10: Twelve Quartz Crystal Reiki Configuration

The Twelve Quartz Crystal Reiki Configurations will enable you to rebalance all the imbalances within the physical, emotional, psychic, and spiritual bodies of one's client.

For this configuration it is always best for your client to be lying on the floor, on some comfortable cushions.

You should position the quartz crystals around your client with one at each point for North, South, East and West and then position two more quartz crystals between each of these points making a full circle around the client. For extra effect the tips or terminations of quartz points can face inward towards the client. (Some can find this energy quite strong, in which case the terminations can be changed to face away from the client).

When your client is comfortable and relaxed you should take your personal control crystal and direct it over all the configuration crystals so that they all become fully energised. You will have then created a powerful electro-magnetic field around your client.

(Charles) *In all my courses, workshops and seminars, and in all my books and writings, I always teach my students and readers that they must use their intuitive faculties in all their treatment sessions: crystal healing and crystal reiki, or, indeed, any other energy-based therapy, should never be done robotically!*

Therefore, while your client is surrounded by powerful crystalline energies, which you will already have programmed to rebalance all the imbalanced energies existing within your client's physical and mental bodies, you can also project your reiki energies to your client at the same time.

Normally I only have my client lying within this configuration for a maximum of forty-five minutes, more often less.

Chapter 11: Crystal Reiki Grid Configurations

Most Crystal Reiki grids, for economic reasons, are created out of copper wiring. The area of your Crystal Reiki copper grid itself should be approximately seven feet x seven feet. In designing your grid, you should interweave the copper wire in such a way that you finish up with spaces two-inches long and seven-inches wide.

The Crystal Reiki copper grid will, obviously, be laid out on the floor. If you or your client find it uncomfortable to lie upon the copper grid itself then I would suggest that you place a white sheet, or robe underneath the body upon which one can lie more comfortably.

While you may lie within this configuration yourself quite safely it is advisable to have someone nearby, perhaps in the next room for safety's sake, as the power and energy created by the Crystal Reiki grid may take you into a very deep and relaxing meditative state, possibly making it difficult to return to normal consciousness.

The Crystal Reiki Copper Grid is a multi-dimensional energy network of immense power.

Copper is a great conductor of energy and by placing double-terminated quartz crystals on the copper grid as shown in the diagram below, all the combined crystalline energy within all the double-terminated quartz crystals is amplified and magnified many times .

You have to experience the effects of the Crystal Reiki Copper Grid for yourself. Words are inadequate to describe all the emotions you will experience or all the subtle energies that you will feel gently pulsating through each level of your innermost being.

As you develop and evolve your spiritual and psychic awareness you will begin to rediscover and remember some of the knowledge and understanding which once was yours when you lived in Atlantis and other important, and relevant, past lifetimes. On occasion it may prove difficult for you to translate this knowledge into words. Our vocabulary simply lacks the words to describe what you are 'seeing' and experiencing, for despite our so-called high-tech civilization and scientific know-how our present-day society still has a very long way to go before it even comes close to the advanced technologies of Atlantis.

Through the Crystal Reiki Copper Grid, you will find that your bodily vibrations will begin to slow down - and become more attuned to the crystalline world around you. Knowledge and understanding will begin to flow from the double-terminated quartz crystals directly into your cosmic consciousness.

And as this information becomes absorbed within your body, at the appropriate time and place you will be able to bring this knowledge and understanding to the surface of your conscious mind to be used for the benefit of the people with whom you are working.

Chapter 12: Animals and Crystal Reiki

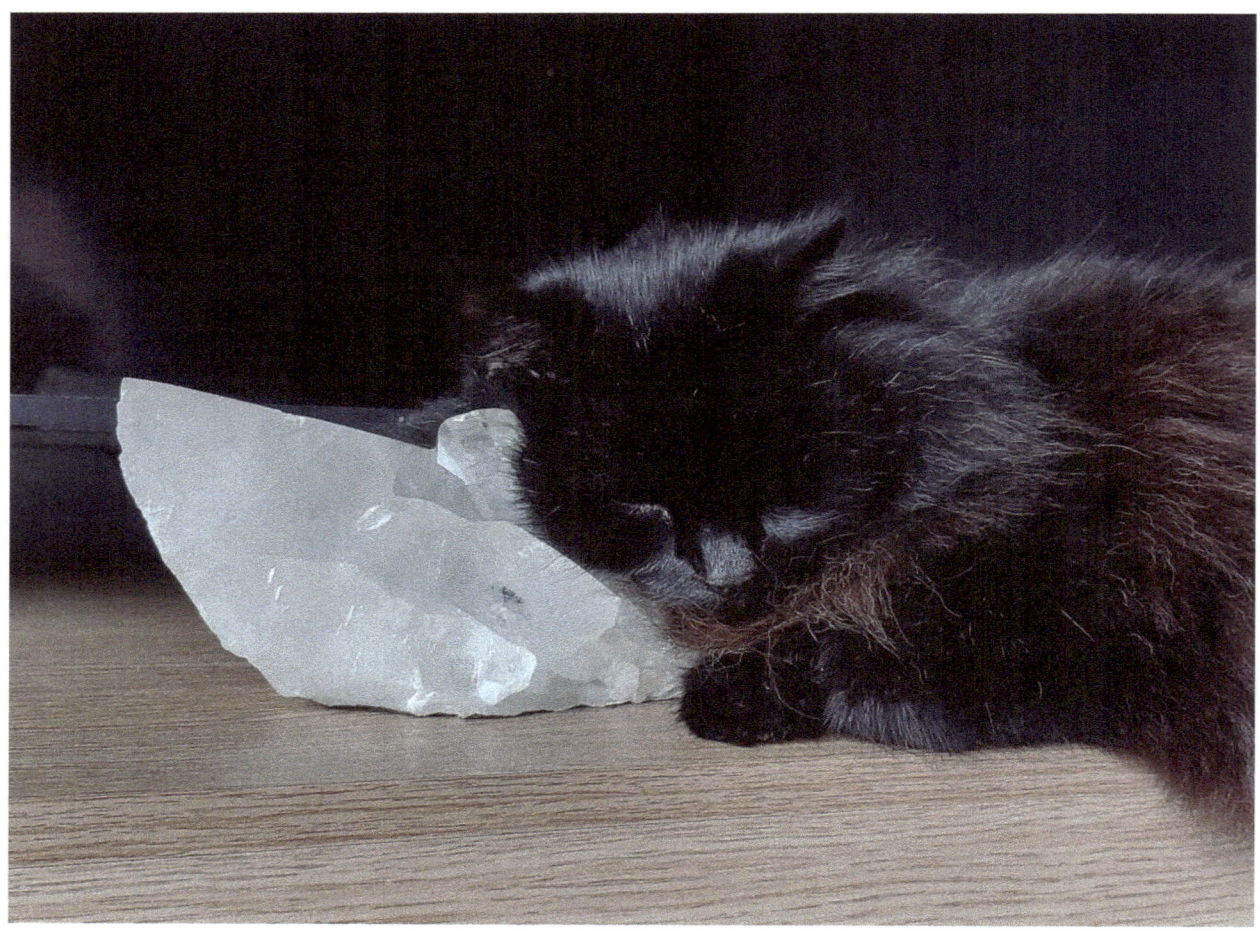

Animals will gravitate towards crystals and their energy and usually lie beside or on them if given the opportunity. They will do this for the duration and amount of time they see fit or for as long is needed.

Lyncara: *It has not been uncommon for me to see animals laying or sleeping on large clusters, particularly Amethyst. It appears, they also approve of its relaxing and sleep inducing properties! I have also seen them lay over or beside a crystal and after a while, move to someone or a client and lay near or beside an area on that person where they have been having issues or symptoms and where healing has been needed. I believe animals heal and give back to us in many ways, and so, it is important to contribute to them and their health in as many ways we can.*

Animals are very in tune to their intuition and perceptions, so it is wise to let the animal decide and choose if they like any crystalline or hands on energies and how long they are around and utilise those energies. Animals know instinctively what they need and they will show us or try to communicate in whatever way they can, especially in reiki energies, where they will usually move and place themselves so your hands are in a certain area to heal. It's important to switch off from thinking too much and thinking like a human, animals do not think and behave like humans although they can feel the same emotions as humans. Allow the animal to communicate to you with body language and allow them to dictate how long their healing session is. Animals are much more receptive than humans and so the process does not always take long at all!

Avoid tying crystals to collars for long periods of time. Some animals are very sensitive to the energies and can become overwhelmed with the weight and the energy of some crystals. If they are strongly affected, they may wish to choose as and when they have access to any crystal energies.

Tying crystals to grate boxes, outside cages or somewhere near the animals bed or safe space is more preferable so the animal can move away if necessary. Always make sure the crystal is stored or tied out of reach of the animal so they can't play, chew or swallow the crystals.

Sometimes, a good way to test a method or a crystals suitability, is to leave different crystals in a safe place, out of reach, where the animal frequently goes and see if the animal responds or prefers any of those energies by being drawn to that area, frequenting the place more often or even sleeping there more. See how they are behaving and responding in those times.

For short sessions of reiki and hands on healing, small, smooth crystals can be used in each hand and placed on or around the body of the animal.

There is no need to add any pressure, just gently brush your hands along the animal in non sensitive places or hold the hands still on or over the area in need of balancing or healing.

Quartz is always a good all round cleanser and healer, sometimes more softer crystalline energies can be useful such as blue chalcedony, morganite, Smokey Quartz, Rose Quartz and moonstones.

Crystals can also be placed around the room, area or table in which the Reiki or Crystal Reiki energy healing is taking place. This way the energies can be used by the therapist or the animal at their own quantum discretion.

Elixirs are a great way to holistically aid in a pets health, however always use the indirect method and leave out the alcohol. In this case, remake the elixir daily as you would change the animals drinking water daily. There is no waste, given the indirect method is using two glass bowls, water in the smallest bowl, placed within the larger bowl which holds the crystal. It can be made in as little as twenty minutes or left overnight for the water to gain the programmed energy from the crystal. Cover the bowls to stop any airbound particles or contamination getting in the water.

NOTE: Never leave crystals in or beside any animal's food or water bowl or trough, or cage no matter how big or small the crystal or the animal!

Never use Crystals and / or Reiki in place of proper veterinary care or medications.

Afterthoughts - Closing statement by Charles.

In many ways, this was a very interesting book for me to write.

I am aware of the fact that although I need to communicate with you using our normal finite terminology, at the same time there is in existence a kind of parallel universal dimension which is continuously exchanging information, ideas and metaphysical thoughts with you at a very deep level within your innermost consciousness.

When you have read this book, I hope that you will have been able to absorb all the hidden teachings which have been programmed within my vibrational words.

This book is written with the intention that you may use it to expand your understanding of, and your capacity to master using crystals with Reiki healing energy. For a more in-depth understanding of the process, I recommend reading my other crystal and gemstone healing books that guide you through the process of using crystal and gemstones in healing therapies.

If you are interested in expanding your knowledge of the healing profession in general, I highly recommend Dr. Patrick Doughtery's excellent book, *Medical Intuition and Muscle Testing*, available on Amazon.

Afterthoughts - Closing statement by Lyncara

After spending so many years in Crystal healing and energy work, it has been a pleasure to share, alongside Charles, some of what I have learned and of the energetic energy and imprints the crystals give to us.

My wish would be for people to grow their intuitive connection to the crystals as devas or living beings in their own right. If we only spend enough time in their vicinity and quieten the mind enough to let them energetically communicate, we can gain so much, not just in knowledge and awareness but in physical energy.

Crystals have been used and carried since the start of man and used in ancient practices and teachings that we are trying to keep alive today. From Atlantis to now, there is much to be said for the technology and information we have regarding crystals. I hope that fellow students and teachers of Crystalline Reiki and other Crystal Arts, continue to think outside the standard limitations and gain more knowledge to share with the world so we may keep the natural teachings of Ancient civilisations and our ancestors alive and progressing.

Chapter 12: Healing Lineage

My Healing Lineage - Charles Lightwalker

Ayurveda Reiki Master: Mohan Chute (founder); Rich Crystal Wolfe; Charles Lightwalker

Activation of the Medicine Wheel
Suzanne Roloff
Charles Lightwalker

Akashic Records
Francine Milford
Zinaid Zeldina
Pamela Jordan
Stephen Lovering
Dori McLean
Wanda Eagleton
Charles Lightwalker

Alchemy Reiki
Suzanne Roloff
Charles Lightwalker

Aloha Reiki, Uhane Nui Reiki & Kahune Reiki Master
Suzanne Roloff
Charles Lightwalker

Ama Deus Shamanic Healing
Guarani
Alberto Aguas
Victor Glanckopf
Michael Arver
Dr. Aurelian Curin
Pamela Jordan
Kavitha Praveen
Yudha Eka Putra
Stephen Lovering
Wanda Eagleton
Charles Lightwalker

Amara Spiritual Empowerment
Omar Antila
Stephen Lovering
Wanda Eagelton
Charles Lightwalker

Ancient Egyptian Healing Modalities

Suzanne Roloff
Charles Lightwalker

Ancient Egyptian Techniques
Suzanne Roloff
Charles Lightwalker

Angel Stones
Suzanne Roloff
Charles Lightwalker

Archangel Michael
Suzanne Roloff
Charles Lightwalker

Archangel Zadkiel Healing System
Rich Crystal Wolfe
Charles Lightwalker

Atlantean Reiki Master
Geoffrey Keytes
Charles Lightwalker

(The) Atlantis Healing System Master
Suzanne Roloff
Charles Lightwalker

Attraction Reiki
Stephanie Brail
Stephen Lovering
Wanda Eagleton
Charles Lightwalker

Blue Star Celestial Energy
Makuan
John Williams
Gary Jirauch
Victor Glanckopf
Dori McLean
Wanda Eagleton
Charles Lightwalker

Celtic Reiki
Martyn Pentacost
Pamela Jordan
Linda Horton
Charles Lightwalker

Celtic Wisdom Energy System
Steve Malcolm
Pamela Jordan
Steve Lovering
Wanda Eagleton
Charles Lightwalker

Crystal Reiki Master
Charles Lightwalker

Crystalline Reiki Master
Charles Lightwalker

Divine Light Reiki
Stephen Comee
Dori McLean
Stephen Lovering
Wanda Eagleton
Charles Lightwalker

Elanari Healing
(Rev) Wendi Wolfwoman Robinson
Charles Lightwalker

Empowerment Reiki
Stephanie Brail
Stephen Lovering
Wanda Eagleton
Charles Lightwalker

(The) Eye of Horus Activation
Suzanne Roloff
Charles Lightwalker

Fusion Reiki
Jason Storm
James McMahon
Dori McLean
Wanda Eagleton
Charles Lightwalker

Hoop Reiki Master
Rich CrystalWolfe
Charles Lightwalker

DNA Reiki
Suzanne Roloff
Charles Lightwalker

Dolphin Heart Reiki
Shanti Johnson
Charles Lightwalker

Elven Shamanic Healing
Suzanne Roloff
Charles Lightwalker

Etheral Crystals
Wanda Ruffner
Shelly Mayer
Dori McLean
Wanda Eagleton
Charles Lightwalker

Fairy Light Raykey
Suzanne Roloff
Charles Lightwalker

Golden Triangle
Isis
James Purner
Linda Vaughn
Dawn Rothwell
Allison Dahlhaus
Wanda Eagleton
Charles Lightwalker

Imara Reiki Master
Barton Wendel
John Vaneekelen
Stephen Womack
Allison Dahlhaus

Inner Light Reiki
Suzanne Roloff
Charles Lightwalker

International Federation of Crystal Healers
Geoffrey Keyte
Charles Lightwalker

Intuitive Emotional Release
Charles Lightwalker

Karuna Ki Reiki
Vincent Amador
Sandra & Jorge Ramos
Allison Dahlhaus
Dori McLean
Kathy McConnell
Charles Lightwalker

Ki Manna
Suzanne Roloff
Charles Lightwalker

Laxmi Reiki
Victor Glanckopf
Dori McLean
Wanda Eagleton
Charles Lightwalker

Imara Reiki Master (cont.)
Dawn Rothwell
Wanda Eagleton
Charles Lightwalker

Karmic Reiki
Mary Pentecost
Pamela Jordan
Claire Timmis
Stephen Lovering
Wanda Eagleton
Charles Lightwalker

Karuna Ki Reiki Master
Vincent Amador
Sandra & Jorge Ramos
Allison Dahlhaus
Wanda Eagleton
Charles Lightwalker

Kundalini Reiki Master
(Rev) Wendi Robinson
Charles Lightwalker

Ma 'heo' o Reiki
Suzanne Roloff
Charles Lightwalker

Medicine Reiki
K'Sitew
Rich CrystalWolf Baker
Charles Lightwalker

Moon Reiki
Suzanne Roloff
Charles Lightwalker

Progressive Healing Techniques
Serena LaSol
Charles Lightwalker

Pyramid, Yod & the Cartouche Mastery
Suzanne Roloff
Charles Lightwalker

Raku-Kei Reiki
Mikao Usul
Chujiro Hayashi Hawayo Takata
Ishikuro
Arthur Robertson
Holly Blackwell
Dori McLean
Stephen Lovering
Wanda Eagleton
Charles Lightwalker

Sacred Flames Reiki Master
Allison Dahlhaus
Charles Lightwalker

Medicine Buddha Reiki
Stephen Cormee
Dori McLean
Shanti Johnson
(Rev) Wendi Robinson
Charles Lightwalker

Orb of Life
Ole Garbrielsen
Victor Glanckopf
Stephen Lovering
Wanda Eagleton
Charles Lightwalker

Pyramid Reiki
Suzanne Roloff
Charles Lightwalker

Sacred Breath Reiki
Wanda Ruffner
Shelly Mayer
Dori McLean
Wanda Eagleton
Charles Lightwalker

Sacred Moon Reiki
Suzanne Roloff
Charles Lightwalker

Sacred Stone Reiki Master

Shanti Johnson
Charles Lightwalker

Seichim Reiki Master
Patrick Zeigler
Tom Seaman
Phoenix Summerfield
Mary Shaw
Christine Henderson
Bruce Way
Ariane McMinn
Frances Wartnaby
Dawn Rothwell
Wanda Eagleton
Charles Lightwalker

Spirit Reiki
Linda Jean Horton
Aroon Kumar
David Paul Benzshawel
Ray Hung
Linda Vaughan
Stephen Lovering
Wanda Eagleton
Charles Lightwalker

Stone Reiki
Suzanne Roloff
Charles Lightwalker

Tibetan Reiki

Tiger Reiki

Tschen Li
Ralph White
Craig Ellis
A. Agee
Light & Adonea
Z. Keyer
Aurellian Curin
C. DiBartolomeo
Linda Horton
Pamela Jordan
Stephen Lovering
Wanda Eagleton
Charles Lightwalker

Stephanie Brail
Stephen Lovering
Wanda Eagleton
Charles Lightwalker

Tree of Life Reiki
Dr. Mikaousui
Dr. Chujiro Hayshi
Hawayo Takata
Phyllis Furumoto
Claudia Hoffman
Mary Shaw
Christine Henderson
Bruce Way
Ariane McMinn
Mona Khalaf
Allison Dahlhaus
Wanda Eagleton
Charles Lightwalker

Violet Flame Reiki
Spirit Kwan Yin
Ivy Moore
Dori McLean
Wanda Eagleton
Charles Lightwalker

White Dove Reiki
Richard Kidd
Dori McLean
Victor Glanckopf
Stephen Lovering
Wanda Eagleton
Charles Lightwalker

Angelic Reiki

Archangel Metatron, KevinCore, Prasthano, Jayn Lee Miller, Cate Akins, Margaret McEwan, Ivan Scott, Angela McGillivray, Charles Lightwalker

Animal Reiki Master Teacher

Charles Lightwalker, Lyncara Stewart

Crystal Healing & Animal Accreditations / Lineage - Lyncara Stewart

Crystal Healing

Crystal Healing and Reflexology Diploma

Crystal and Hot Stone Therapy Diploma

Animal Communication and Healing Diploma - Karen E Wells, Lyncara A Stewart

Animal Reiki Diploma

Animal Reiki Master Teacher

Animal Kinesiology Diploma

Animal Anatomy and physiology B.A Hons

Equestrian Care / Anatomy and physiology Diploma

Pure Energy Crystal Healing - Mark Bajerski, Lyncara A Stewart

Angelic Reiki levels 1 & 2 - Marilyn Harris, Lyncara A Stewart

Usui Reiki - Alison Simpson, Lyncara A Stewart

Tuning Forks Practitioner, Charles Lightwalker, Lyncara A Stewart

Medical Intuitive Practitioner

Shamanism Rites of the Munay Ki

Animal Cosmology

Reiki Resources

The Following organisations support Reiki professionals and offer an opportunity to network with other Reiki practitioners throughout the world. I have been a member of several of these professional organisations and continue to support their efforts to educate the public and to increase the awareness of Reiki in the world, so that we all may feel and experience the healing energy of Reiki.

International Reiki Organization

reikiassociation.com

International Reiki Healing Association

reikihealingassociation.com

Reiki Therapy Resources

reikitherapyresources.com

International Association of Reiki Professionals

iarp.org

The Reiki Association

reikiassociation.net

Reiki

reiki.org

Reiki Association of America

reikiasociationofamerica.com

American International Reiki Association

reikiview.com

Reiki Healing association

www.reikihealingassociation.com

Angelic Reiki International

www.angelicreikiinternational.com

Angelic Reiki Association

www.angelicreikiassociation.com

Angelic Reiki UK

https:angelicreikiuk.com

This is the list so far, if there are other reiki organisations, please email us and we will add it to our list of resources with thanks. Charles.

ABOUT - Charles Lightwalker

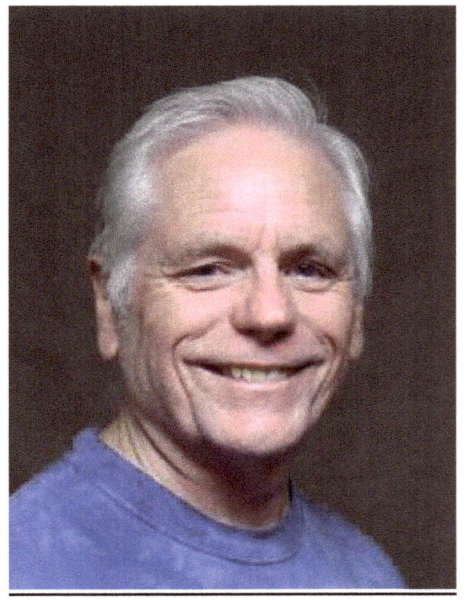

Charles Lightwalker is a writer, poet, dreamer, storyteller, teacher, healer, and visionary, and holds a PhD In Shamanism/Religious Studies, a Master's degree in Chaplaincy studies, and is a nondenominational minister. Charles also is a shamanic practitioner/teacher, certified Religious Counsellor, Certified Spiritual Healer, Reiki Master/Teacher, and loves dancing, taking walks, riding his bicycle, doing meditation and yoga.

Charles is a member of the following organisations, The Foundation for Shamanic Studies Council member, Society of Shamanic Practitioners, Spokane Holistic Chamber of Commerce, Spokane Metaphysical Research Society, Vietnam Veterans of America, and serves on the board of directors of the International Association of Medical Intuitives. He is also an elder on the council of the Cherokee Wolf Clan of the Pacific Northwest. Charles is also the co-author of *Quantum Healing: The Synergy of Chiropractic* and *Reiki; Medical Intuition and Muscle Testing,* and author of *Whip Flash Soup and other Spiritual Ingredients,* a book of poetry. Charles is writing two more books currently, an autobiography and *Musings: A Collection of Writings*.

ABOUT: Lyncara Aria Stewart

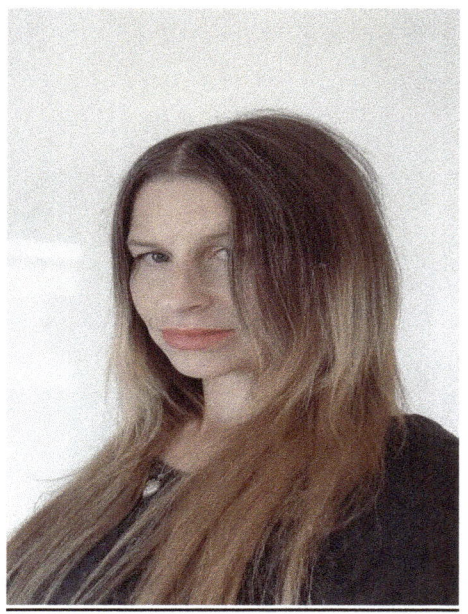

Lyncara is an Animal Communicator and an Animal Reiki Master Teacher, using Reiki, Kinesiology and Crystals to bring comfort to all animals. She has worked with crystals and their healing properties for over 30 years. She is also certified in many other healing modalities, including Crystal Healing and Reflexology, Reiki, Energy Healing, Medical Intuition, Tuning forks, Animal care, Animal Anatomy and Physiology, Colour therapy, Water therapy, Shamanism and has also started her journey into the realm of being an author to share the findings of her work with Crystals and Healing work.

Her passion started at a very young age with a love for animals and crystals, leading her to where she is today and ever acquiring more knowledge. She enjoys the old shamanic teachings of ceremony and healing and partakes in sharing Animal Cosmology in her intuitive readings so others can learn to connect to the animals, their spirit and their teachings.

Lyncara spends her time immersed in nature any time she can, a lover of the beach she can be found there surfing, fossil and crystal hunting, barefoot walking, painting, reading or writing a book, taking photographs of nature, animals and crystals. She likes to go waterfall hunting and wild swimming, enjoying remote places and time in the wild either by foot or by riding her motorcycle.

Lyncara is a member of the International Association of Medical Intuitives and is continuing to write books on her workings and findings with crystals, crystal skulls, energy healing and working with animals and people on physical and quantum levels.

A Reiki Glossary of Terms

A

Adama Star Fire Reiki: A form of Reiki energy that is channelling to the Earth from the stars

Ai-Reiki: The state of being in harmony with Reiki

Angelic Ray Key (Reiki): A healing discipline for the twenty-first century. The focus is on healing and uplifting all areas of living: body, mind, and spirit

Anshin Ritsumei (also: Dai Anjin): A state in which one's mind is totally at peace, and not bothered by anything. A state in which one perceives one's life's purpose

Ascension Reiki: A method of opening up to the great outpouring of divine love

B

Brahma Satya Reiki: An evolution of the spiritual descent of Shiva-Shakti in the form of Brahma Satya

Byosen Reikan-ho: Also simply called *Byosen*. A Reiki technique for sensing energetic fluctuations

C

Chakra Kassei Kokyo-ho: A chakra-activating breathing method

Celtic Reiki: A form of Reiki discovered by Martyn Pentecost of Croydon U.K. which employs symbols derived from the Celtic ogham (the ancient alphabet used by the Druids)

Choku Rei: The name of the first of the four Usui Reiki symbols. Commonly called the "Power" symbol in Takata-lineage Reiki (Usui Shiki Ryoho). In Japanese lineages the symbol is commonly called the `Focus' symbol' [some relate it to the earth element]. Takata-Sensei translated Choku Rei as "put the [spiritual] power here," yet it can also translate as something akin to: "in the direct presence of Spirit"

Crystal Reiki: A form of reiki developed by Charles Lightwalker

Crystalline Reiki: A form of reiki founded during meditation by shamanic reiki master Charles Lightwalker

D

Dai Ko Myo: The name of the last of the four Usui Reiki symbols. Commonly called the `Master' symbol in Takata-lineage Reiki (Usui Shiki Ryoho). The ` symbol' is actually the words Dai, Ko, & Myo written in kanji, and name literally means: `Great Shining Light,' signifying `Enlightened Nature' or `the Radiant Light of Wisdom,' the Radiance of a Deity (Buddha, Bodhisattva, `Vidyaraja', etc), or the manifest expression of the Light of Wisdom: the means by which illumination "dawns on us"

Denju: 'Initiation'- the `Western' style Reiki attunement process used by Takata-Sensei

Divine Light Reiki: A new system based on the Japanese system Jôrei, or Johrei, that was developed in the early twentieth century by Mokichi Okada, founder of the Church of World Messianity

Dragon Reiki: A form of reiki developed by Victor Glanckopf

Dolphin Reiki: A form of reiki developed by Shanti Johnson

E

Eguchi te-no-hira Ryoji: A hand/palm healing modality developed by Toshihiro Eguchi (a friend and student of Usui Sensei), said to incorporate elements of Usui-do Enkaku Chiryo-Ho `Distant Healing Method'
Excalibur reiki: A system of reiki in which you attune to the energy of Excalibur, the Sword of Truth as well as the archetypal energies of Merlin and the Lady of the Light to heal and manifest

F

G

Gakkai: A "Learning Society," such as the Usui Reiki Ryoho

Gakkai Gassho: A ritual gesture formed by placing the hands together in a prayer-like position in front of the mouth, and the fingertips at a level just below the nose. "Gassho" implies recognition of the oneness of all beings. This gesture is also used to show reverence to Buddhas, Bodhisattvas, Patriarchs & Teachers of Gassho Kokyu-Ho

Gassho Breathing Method: The practice of `breathing' through the hands while in the Gassho position

Gassho Meiso: Gassho Meditation

Gendai Reiki Ho: Modern Reiki Method. A modern form of Japanese Reiki created by Hiroshi Doi, combining some traditional Usui teachings and techniques with teachings and techniques from other energy-healing arts

Gendoku-Ho: A detoxification technique in which one hand is placed at *seika tanden*, the other on the lower back at approximately the same level

Gold Reiki : While there is not much information available on Gold Reiki, it is considered to be very powerful Reiki of the Gold Ray. It transmutes fear and darkness into light and joy! Gold Light is the strongest light of transformation in the physical universe! The Gold Ray is a very purifying energy

Gokai: The Five Reiki Principles / Precepts Gokai Sansho Recitation of the Five Reiki Principles / Precepts (sansho here refers to `three times')

Grandmaster Reiki: A termed used by Charles Lightwalker and other Reiki Practitioners that denotes the creator of a Reiki form

Gyosei: Poetry penned by the Meiji Emperor, about 125 of which are recited at meetings of the Usui Reiki Ryoho Gakkai. [These poems are in a style known as waka]

Gyoshi-Ho: "Gazing Method," a technique of healing with the eyes

H

Hado Kokyu-Ho: A breathing technique, said to raise ones vibrational levels

Hado Meiso: Ho Hado-breath meditation

Hanshin Chiryo-Ho: `Half-body Treatment Method'

Hanshin Koketsu-Ho: 'Half-body Blood-purifying Method'

Hara: 'Belly:' the extended area between the top of the pubic bone and the base of the sternum

Hatsurei Ho: Initiate (*Hatsu*) Spirit (*Rei*) Method (*Ho*); a set of primarily *Ki-jutsu* techniques which Usui Sensei is said to have taught as an aid to self-development

Heso Chiryo-Ho: Acupressure-type energy-balancing technique applied to the navel with middle finger

Hibiki: 'Reverberation;' sensation in the hands, the nature of which can indicate the presence and status of a dis-ease

Hikari no Kokyu-Ho 'Breath of Light' Method; a variant of *Joshin Kokyo-Ho*

Hikkei: A handbook or manual

Hon Sha Ze Sho Nen: Name of the third of the four Usui Reiki symbols. Commonly called the 'distant' symbol in Takata-lineage Reiki (*Usui Shiki Ryoho*). This ' symbol' is actually the words: Hon, Sha, Ze, Sho, &Nen, written in kanji (albeit in a stylised form). While some people have sought to translate the phrase 'Hon Sha Ze Sho Nen' as: "no past, no present, no future", this mantra phrase actually translates as: 'True mindfulness is the source of essential being.' It does not represent an energy, but a state of mind, a connectedness to all things

Holy Fire Reiki: Developed by William Lee Rand

I

Imara Reiki: An advanced reiki level beyond Reiki Master. Imara is incredibly powerful, yet it does not need symbols. Imara is recognized as Level V on the Reiki energy scale that some people use. Imara Reiki uses a new and easy attunement process. Barton Wendel first channelled Imara

In-Yo: Japanese equivalent of the Chinese Yin-Yang

J

Jaki Kiri Joka Ho: AtTechnique for 'energetic cleansing' of inanimate objects. NOT to be used on living things: people, plants or animals [This technique seems to be derived from a more involved practice called the `Ki Barai']

Jikiden Reiki: `Original Teaching' or `Directly Taught' Reiki; Japanese Reiki as taught by Chiyoko Yamaguchi, a student of Chujiro Hayashi.

Joshin Kokyo-Ho: Cleansing Breathing technique used to stimulate, strengthen and purify the flow of Reiki; a component of

Jumon: A Mantra or Sacred Invocation

K

Kaicho: A president / chairman; title of the Leader of The Usui Reiki Ryoho Gakkai

Kanji: Chinese characters used for writing Japanese

Kanboku: A term used to indicate the Reiki symbols by Yuji Onuki, a student of Toshihiro Eguchi [see also *shirushi*]

Kantoku: Illuminating visionary mystical state; brought about by practice of strict ascetic mystical disciplines including fasting, isolation, meditation & the use of incantation and mudra-like techniques

Karmic Reiki: A style of Reiki style created by Martyn Pentecost, which although based on Usui Reiki techniques, is used in a slightly different manner in order to deal with the various issues that arise from negative karmic events

Karuna Reiki: Karuna is a Sanskrit word for compassion and is used in Hinduism and Buddhism. Developed by William Rand

Karuna Ki: An advanced form of Reiki developed by Vincent Amador.

Kenyoku-Ho: `Dry Brushing Method' - essentially an aura-cleansing technique - a component of *Hatsurei-Ho*

Ketsueki Kokan-Ho: The Reiki `Finishing' or `Smoothing' technique

Ki-jutsu: `Energetic Arts' - Collective term for Japanese disciplines concerned with the development, strengthening and refinement of `Ki'

Ki Ko: Japanese name for the Chinese Art of Chi Gung (Qi Gong)

Kiriku: The `spiritual emblem' of Amida Butsu, and probable origin of the second of the four Usui Reiki symbols - Sei Heiki

Koketsu-Ho:`Blood-purifying Method' Koki-Ho `Exhalation (Koki) Method' - technique of healing with the breath Kokoro Heart, Spirit, Will or Mind

Kokyo-Ho: Breathing Techniques for Development, Strengthening and Purification of *Ki Koshin-do Mawashi*, the `Reiki Circle' method. [also called *Reiki Mawashi*]

Kotodama: 'Word-Spirit,' a Shinto practice involving the intonation of individual syllables and vowel-sounds

Kouki: With Zenki, one of the two inner levels comprising Okuden, the second level of Reiki training.

Kundalini Reiki: A method founded by Ole Gabrielsen

Kurama Yama: Horse-saddle (Kurama) Mountain (Yama); the Sacred Mountain where Usui-Sensei is believed to have first experienced Reiki [though some have suggested Mount Koya as the original site]

L

Laxmi Reiki: Lakshmi or Laxmi is the Hindu goddess of Wealth, fortune and luck.
Lavender Flame of Quan Yin: A fraction of the Violet Flame of Transmutation.

Light Dream Reiki: A method channelled in 2003 by Alla Sharkia. Light Dream Reiki works well for those suffering from insomnia. There are no symbols in this method and this is highest frequency based on the power of the Violet Ray of St. Germain

Lunar Light Reiki Empowerment: Developed by the Founder of Kundalini Reiki, Ole Gabrielsen

M

Makoto No Kokyu: A Hara Defining Exercise contained in the two inner levels of Okuden (*Zenki* & *Kouki*), being one of many different meditations and energy exercises taught at these levels. This is a very powerful meditation and has been practised in Japan since the 8th century, but it is much older, probably about 2000 years old.

Medicine Buddha Reiki: a well-known healing practice, with roots in the Mahayana Buddhist tradition.

N

Nade-Te Chiryo-Ho: Stimulating the flow of ki in the body by stroking with the hand

Nentatsu-Ho: Form of `thought-transmission' via the hands

O

Okuden: Level II in some versions of the Reiki Grading system

Oshite Chiryo-Ho: `Pressing Hand', actually, an acupressure-type technique applied with the fingertips

P
Q
R

Raku Kei Reiki: The words Rei-Ki originate from the words Raku-Kei. It is thought to have been a forerunner of Reiki and incorporates the Fire element of breathing used to increase the energy of Reiki. Raku-Kei is the ancient science of Self-development and Self-improvement

Ra-Sheeba Reiki: Founded by Merilyn Bretherick and Peter Johansen of Victoria, Australia, Ra-Sheeba incorporates creative sexual energy (Sheeba) with veneration of the solar source (Ra)

Rei: To Bow; as in: *Kamiza ni Rei* [bow to the Altar], *Otagai ni Rei* [bow to fellow students], *Sensei (Gata) ni Rei* [bow to ones teacher(s)], *Shinzen ni Rei* [bow to a shrine.], *Ritsu* (or *Tachi*) *Rei* [standing bow], *Za Rei* [kneeling bow]. By bowing, you are expressing respect, courtesy, and gratitude to your art, your sensei, dojo (training establishment), other students, and yourself [This `rei' is not written in the same kanji as the `rei' in `Reiki']

Reiho: Etiquette; a method of bowing

Reiho: `Spiritual Method;' as in: Usui Reiho: Usui Spiritual Method Some people claim that `Reiho' is a contraction of: `Reiki Ryoho' (Reiki Healing Method) This `Reiho' is not written in the same kanji as the `Reiho' meaning Etiquette] Reiji `Indication of the Spirit' - Spiritual guidance in the placing of your hands to give treatment

Reiju Spiritual (Rei) Gift (Ju); term for the original form of Reiki Attunement-Empowerment

Reiki: The term commonly used to indicate the therapeutic and self-development system created by Mikao Usui, and more specifically, the wonderful therapeutic energy radiance, or phenomenon, which lies at the heart of this natural healing system. The word `Reiki' has, it seems, achieved generic status, being used to refer to numerous hands-on healing practices of unrelated origin. Reiki can translate as: `Spiritual Energy', `Spiritual Feeling,' and in some instances can be used as a term for an Ancestral Spirit

Reikika A Reiki Practitioner

`*Reiki Ryoho No Shion*': (Kind Teacher's Reiki Method of Healing) - the title of a Reiki manual said to be given to all members of the Usui Reiki Ryoho Gakkai

Reiki Un-do A method of Reiki treatment received through spontaneous movement; albeit intentionally initiated

Renzoku: A `Reiki marathon'

Ryoho: 'Healing Method; Medical Treatment;' as in *Usui Reiki Ryoho*: Usui Reiki Healing Method

S

Sacred Flames Reiki (SFR) is a powerful system compiled by Allison Dahlhaus from different resources (in the physical and spiritual realms) to share with all those drawn to it. SFR is a set of guided visualisations and meditations designed to help the body, mind, and spirit heal themselves, and/or to maintain good balance within the systems of the body, both physically and energetically.

Saibo Kassei Ka: A cell-activating technique

Seichim, (pronounced say-keem), is an Egyptian word meaning power. It was discovered in 1984 by an American Reiki Master, Patrick Zeigler, much in the same mystical way as Dr. Usui received Reiki

Seiheki Chiryo-Ho: A variant form of *Nentatsu-Ho Sei Heiki*. The second of the four Usui Reiki symbols: commonly called the 'mental/emotional' symbol in Takata-lineage Reiki (*Usui Shiki Ryoho*). In Japanese lineages the symbol is commonly called the 'Harmony' symbol' [some relate it to the water element]. Depending on the kanji used to write 'Sei Heiki', the name can mean 'emotional calmness' or 'spiritual composure'

Seiza: Traditional Japanese kneeling posture, sitting back on (or between) the heels

Sekizui Joka Ibuki-Ho: Spinal Cord (*Sekizui*) Purification (*Joka*) Breath (*Ibuki*) Method (*Ho*); a technique of 'insufflation' or blowing of energy-breath to release negativity from the spine

Shiki: 'Style'- as in *Usui Shiki Ryoho*: Usui Style Healing Method

Shinpiden: Level III (Master Level) in some versions of the Reiki Grading system

Shirushi: 'Symbol'

Shoden: Level III in some versions of the Reiki Grading system

Shu Chu Reiki: Reiki Treatment given to a single individual by a group

Spirit Reiki: A system of spirit growth and healing that is available to Usui Reiki Masters. This system uses two Usui Reiki symbols as well as four additional symbols that were given to Linda Jean Horton

Sufi Reiki: A form of reiki that takes healing to the next level, empowering the individual to move beyond an awakening and toward self-realisation.

T

Tibetan Reiki: is a system of energy healing that helps to bring our energies into balance and harmony.

Tanden Chiryo-Ho: A body detoxification technique

Te-Ate: 'Hand-Treatment' - generic term for Japanese hands-on healing modalities

U

Uchite Chiryo-Ho: A Shiatsu-like patting or palpating technique

Usui: A term used by many Japanese shamanic practitioners to describe 'power spots;' places where the 'veil' between this world and the World of the Spirit is thin. It should be stressed that the Japanese word, *usui*, meaning thin, while a synonym for the surname of Usui sensei, is written in different kanji than the founder's name and is not related to it.

Usui Do: 'Usui's Way'. Term used to refer to Usui-sensei's original system of Spiritual Development

Usui Reiki Ryoho: 'Usui Reiki Healing Method.' Term used to refer to Reiki as it evolved in Japan. Said to be closer to Usui-Sensei's original format, it uses *reiju* rather than the symbol-centred attunements familiar in 'western' style Reiki

Usui Reiki Ryoho Gakkai: (Usui Reiki Healing Method Learning Society). While some say the society was founded by Usui-Sensei himself in 1922, it is generally accepted that the Gakkai was actually founded by Rear Admiral Juusaburo Gyuda (Ushida) and other students around 1926

Usui Shiki Ryoho: 'Usui Style Healing Method'. 'Western' Reiki as taught by Takata-Sensei -a system divided into three levels, using attunements involving the four Reiki symbols

Usui Teate: 'Usui Hand Treatment'. Term used by some of Usui-Sensei's surviving students to refer to his Healing Method.

V

Violet Flame Reiki: a form of Reiki using the violet flame as part of the healing process.

W

Waka: 'Japanese Song.' Short poems with lines containing fixed numbers of syllables, traditionally 5-7-5-7-7. The familiar haiku of 5-7-5 syllable lines are an abbreviated form of *waka*

White Dove Reiki™ Although there are many forms of Reiki, White Dove Reiki™ enables the Reiki Practitioner to have assistance in the Healing and Attunement process.

X

Y

Yagyu Ryu: Usui Sensei is believed to have achieved the high ranking of `Menkyo Kaiden' in *Yagyu Ryu*, a *Bujutsu* (Martial Arts) School focusing on the arts of *Kenjutsu* (sword-fighting) & *Ju-jutsu* (unarmed combat) - founded by Yagyu Muneyoshi Tajima no Kami (1527-1606).

Z

Zenki: With *Kouki*, one of the two inner levels comprising *Okuden*, the second level of Reiki training.

Zenshin Koketsu-Ho: Full-body Treatment Method

Final Afterthought - Charles

Putting together this manual and then revising it with Lyncara, has been a lot of fun, and has given me the opportunity to relearn some of my forgotten Reiki terms, some of my Reiki background has rekindled my interest in the art of Reiki as a healing modality. It has guided me to take an Angelic Reiki Course in Scotland from Angela McGillivray, and to also take an Animal Reiki Course, given by the Reiki Healing Association headquartered in the United Kingdom.

This adventure has led me to realise I want to get back into teaching again, especially the medical intuition practitioner certification course I taught in America. I also have been excited to get back into my Metis Medicine Ways teaching, and share the knowledge.

Moving to Scotland has been one of the best things that I have done in my life, walking on the beach and feeling the raw nature of Scotland, and adjusting my life to new adventures, new opportunities, and making new friends. What a blessing it has been.

Charles.

Final Afterthought - Lyncara

It has been a pleasure to co-author this book with Charles. He has so much knowledge and experience to share with the world and it is obvious it is his passion and keenness to do so. Charles is always expanding his knowledge and connecting others into the realm of spirit and community.

Learning and upgrading my reiki to Animal Master Teacher with Charles as my teacher has been a blessing and putting those years of crystal healing experience with people and animals to use within this book made sense and is an honour to do so, not just alongside my mentor but to share this information and knowledge with the world and like minded people and practitioners.

I have dedicated my life to being a voice to the animals and to bring awareness back to the natural ways that have been used over centuries and from ancient times, so that we can be connected to the earth, spirit and ourselves. To better our physical, spiritual and emotional health, especially in today's modern world. It is a service to spirit, the ancestors and the ancients that came before us.

It is my hope, this kind of work continues and evolves over time, with more practitioners leading the way of homeostasis and equilibrium for physical, emotional and spiritual health and happiness for humans and animals alike. That we remember and feel our connection to the cosmos, to life, to earth, to the cycle, to our ancestors and to the divine.

Lyncara.

Closing statement

This book has been a long process, that began in 2002, when my child River was born, becoming a father made me look at the future, the world around me and how I could empower my child to survive in a world with political corruption and environmental chaos.

Bringing this book to completion would not have happened without the help of Lyncara, a crystal and gemstone expert, who could see the value of the book and encouraged me to redo it, revise it and rethink it, and republish it . Lyncara's input and contributions have made this book more complete.

Lyncara has added a depth to this manuscript that it was lacking. Her gifts as an Animal Reiki Master teacher, crystal healer, Animal communicator, and devotion to being of service to her clients, with integrity and honesty has renewed my hope for the future of the healing arts. She is the next generation of Master healers to help humankind.   June 2024

Charles.

www.ingramcontent.com/pod-product-compliance
Lightning Source LLC
Chambersburg PA
CBHW051316110526
44590CB00031B/4371